CW00971624

# A GUT FE
# PROBIOTIC
# SMOOTHIES

## TO CLEANSE-HEAL-ENERGISE & LOSE WEIGHT

101+ Delicious Recipes For Gut Health.

Green Smoothie Drinks, Power foods - Recipes and 10 day cleanse plan. Using a mix of fruit, vegetables and super foods with Probiotics. Discover how these are instrumental in a healthy successful cleanse and a healthy diet.

© 2015 printBook 1st edition xii.i.xv.

VALLEY RIDGE PRESS.

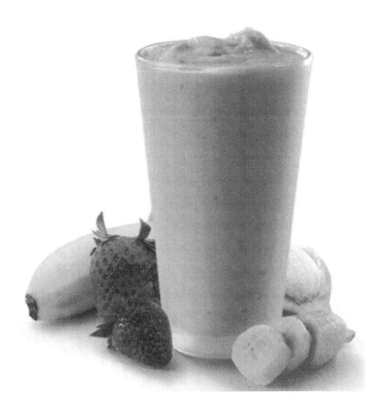

## *It's simple!*

*Every, and YES! I mean EVERY Successful detox and healthy smoothie cleanse plan, should start with probiotic recipes. These recipes feed and establish good bacteria back in to your gut. Then you can introduce recipes high in prebiotic to top up and feed your good bacteria. Now your body can successfully absorb the minerals, vitamins and phytonutrients you consume in your smoothies.*

A Gut Feeling Probiotic Smoothies.

To Cleanse-Heal-Energize & Lose Weight.

© 2015 by VALLEY RIDGE PRESS.

Printed in the USA

Learn more information at: Oliver Michaels Author on AMAZON.

Follow The Author on Real Healthy Kinda Food on Facebook for up to date information and recipes. Real healthy kinda living.

# TABLE OF CONTENTS

**Chapter 5**

The miracle Water Cure

**Chapter 6**

Now Lets start the 3-10 day detox cleanse

Day 1 - 10. One day at a time

**Chapter 7**

101 Recipes for Health and Vitality.

Detoxification Smoothies

Diabetes/blood sugar control Smoothies

Energy Pre workout Smoothies

Healthy heart Smoothies

Boosting your Immunity Smoothies

Kid friendly Recipes Smoothies

Stress beater Smoothies

Fat burner Smoothies

Mood enhancing Smoothies

Pregnancy / Kid friendly smoothies

Constipation Smoothies

Healing strong bones and joints Smoothies

# DEDICATION

For Luca x

Also, to all who have suffered from the food industries greed and their lack of any nutritional content in our modern food. May this book and all the delicious recipes serve as a healthy power smoothie remedy to us all.

# EPIGRAPH
## "ALL DISEASE BEGINS IN THE GUT " ~ HIPPOCRATES

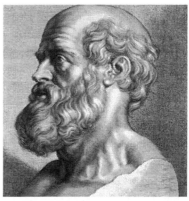

It has been over two thousand years since Hippocrates made this bold statement; it has never been as true or relevant as it is today. Our digestive tract is the passageway through one end of the body to the other. For the most part, it provides a barrier between the outside world and our insides. It's only through the digestive process involving specialized cells that the nutrients from food actually enter the body. Any disruption in the health, function, or interaction of these cells with each other or their environment can significantly compromise not only the absorption of nutrients but also our overall health.

Medical historians will generally look to Hippocrates as the founder of medicine as a rational science. It was in fact Hippocrates who finally freed medicine from the shackles of magic, superstition, and the supernatural.

He collected data and conducted experiments to show that disease was a natural process. He also discovered that the signs and symptoms of a disease were caused by the natural reactions of the body to the disease process, and that the chief role of the physician was to aid the natural resistance of the body to overcome the metabolic imbalance and restore health and harmony to the organism.

# ABOUT THE AUTHOR.

Congratulations for taking control of your health. The best investment of your life…

Oliver Michaels was born in Newcastle England, in 2009 he moved to North America where he now lives with his family. He is a best selling author, avid reader, thinker, husband, doer', and a loving dad.

He is a highly dedicated foodie, passionate and enthusiastic about his own and his family's future health and diet. He is strongly committed to investigative research, writing, publishing and creative marketing.

Oliver's focus is on writing compelling and alternative information on his investigative research and passion of healthy foods and healthy living.

The quotes he is most driven and inspired by are: -

"I have NOT failed... I have just found 10,000 ways that won't work..." Thomas Edison.

"People will forget what you said, People will forget what you did, but people will never forget how you made them feel." Maya Angelou.

"Imagination is more important than knowledge". Albert Einstein.

Oliver claims to have read just about every healthy diet and marketing book out there, and he still gets inspired and learns something new every day.

His work ethic is on continual improvement, investigative research and creative thinking.

Every Month Oliver gives away thousands of his eBooks through amazon kindle worldwide. It is his goal to share his research and discoveries with everyone who is like-minded and especially passionate about food and healthy living.

Email Oliver directly at: -

olivermichaels.author@hotmail.com if you have any questions or for more information.

# WHY *I* WROTE THIS BOOK.

*"...I want to share my research and recipes with like-minded people who are driven and want to vastly improve their health and wellness. Most of all I want to share my experiences and journey during my research to give you sustained health and happiness.*

Since the age of 11 years old I have suffered with abdominal pains and poor digestion. In later years I was diagnosed with I.B.S along with millions of other sufferers worldwide. The symptom of my I.B.S was inflammation, severe abdominal cramps, severe bloating, nausea and rosacea.

In May 2011, my son Luca was born in the UK. He was just perfect and so beautiful, *as all babies are.* ☺.

After we returned to our home in Canada, we made a visit to our family doctor and introduced Luca to her. After a week and some tests later Luca was found to have acute lactose intolerance. Oh well, I having suffered years from inflammation was also tested where I was also diagnosed with lactose intolerance.

Our son Luca grew steadily and healthy meeting all his milestones, he was growing and developing fast. He then reached the age of 18 months. He had just received his vaccinations and then suffered from a bad pneumonia. This went undiagnosed for over 5 weeks, despite our daily calls, visits and pleas with the doctors at urgent care pleading he was unwell.

*As a parent you just know something is wrong, 'a gut feeling', despite a "medical professional" saying otherwise.*

After Luca slowly got over his pneumonia there was a noticeable decline in his development. After one year and many psychologists meetings, consultations and testing, our worst

11

fears were confirmed. Luca was diagnosed with ASD, (autism Spectrum disorder).

Anyone who has gone through this will understand it is like having all your hopes and dreams for your baby crushed. Then you are left with a huge empty void, your mind constantly being filled with questions.

We were both deeply grieving, while still trying to provide support and care for Luca. It was a long continuous roller coaster of emotions from initial anger, denial and then disbelief. All was re-presenting itself to us in an ever-changing weekly cycle.

We eventually found ourselves resting at the doors of hope. Our hope was we could make Luca's life as full filling and happy as possible. We needed to find normality for Luca that we feared he would never have.

Several years earlier, I had heavily researched and discovered juicing cleansing and the paleo diet. This diet totally alleviated my stomach issues and allowed me to recover from my many symptoms of continual stomach inflammation and severe pain.

Lisa and I now live and enjoy a healthy life we are 100% Paleo, about 80% of the time.

At the age of two, I decided to introduce Luca to my green juice supplements. He seemed to thrive on these healthy organic juice recipes. It was here I saw small glimpses of hope.

I strongly support areas of medical research that backup *'our gut health and the links to all ailments, our brain function and development'*.

The fact is Luca just couldn't get enough of the juice. We saw glimpses of change in his development and behavior. We then began to cut out ALL wheat and gluten from his diet.

I knew through my years of reading and investigative research into my I.B.S and now my son's autism, there was a link between our modern diet, our brain and our gut health.

Conditions including metabolic syndrome, inflammatory bowel disease, obesity, rheumatoid arthritis, depression, chronic fatigue syndrome and autism spectrum disorder.

To be honest I continue to see so much of myself in my son Luca. There are so many similarities. I too had a Speech delay - I've suffered food intolerance most my life – I had early learning and concentration issues all throughout my schooling. One similarity all children with A.S.D have is, they ALL suffer diet limitations, food allergies and/or food intolerance.

Who was it said all disease begins in the gut…?

The realisation and the belief having read and researched many great medical documents have led me to release this book.

Today, Luca is developing faster than we could have hoped. He is continuing to show some amazing signs of development and improvement. Despite him being pre-verbal he has made significant steps where the *hope* of Luca reaching a successful independent future is getting near to a reality.

So that's why I'm here in front of you now, whether you want to lose weight, suffer from inflammation, food allergies, intolerance, colitis, bloating, or you just want a quick healthy cleanse diet, then this book will tick all your boxes.

I strongly believe in hope, and I'm on constant pursuit for continual improvement, I never stop looking for answers. This book is dedicated to Luca, and all of you who have joined me in this approach to drink healthy green smoothies and focus on their gut health.

13

EVERY! Successful detox and healthy cleanse plan should start with probiotic Smoothie recipes. The probiotic recipes, through the fibers, feed and establish good bacteria back into your gut. You can then introduce recipes high in prebiotics and phytonutrients to top up and feed the good bacteria.

Only now do we successfully concentrate on improving our health with a Smoothie cleanse.

After re-establishing your gut health your body will be highly efficient in absorbing all the vitamins, minerals and phytonutrients you try to get throughout your day. You will alleviate hunger as the bad bacteria no longer dominate and send messages to your brain through your enteric nervous system, craving more food.

The Probiotic Smoothie Recipe Book provides you with a host of major health information, recipes and benefits…

# QUICK START

OK, so you want to drink your way to incredible health and enjoy tasty smoothies made with your new blender, starting right NOW! To start here is a collection of three recipes for those on the go busy people who just want to get right into it. I have given you a choice of three quick, easy and delicious recipes you can just throw into your blender and voila... You have a delicious tasting healthy smoothie. There are over 100+ incredible recipes in chapter 6.

### 1. Blueberry & Banana Smoothie

2 handfuls greens

1-cup water

1 large banana, peeled and frozen

1 1/4 cups frozen blueberries

¼ cup ground flaxseeds

1 packet stevia (to sweeten – Optional)

### 2. Strawberry & Green Smoothie ⊕

2 handfuls greens

1/2-cup green tea

½ cups frozen strawberries

1 banana, peeled and frozen

1 packet stevia

15

**Banana & Pear Smoothie**

2 handfuls greens

11/2 cups water

1 banana, peeled and frozen

2 pears cored and seeded

2 tablespoons ground chia seed

⊕ = GOOD PREBIOTICS

Also <u>(See paragraph 7)</u> For all 101+ Smoothie recipes.

# CHAPTER 1

## FOCUS ON YOUR GUT HEALTH.

Before we start making even more smoothies, please read on to fully understand the incredible health benefits of drinking smoothies every day. You will find delicious healthy recipes, benefits and power foods supplements for you to discover. You can start making smoothies with your new blender and include these in your daily diet routine.

We need to focus on our gut health and how we can incorporate ingredients that are rich in phytonutrients and very tasty.

Do you want to know why getting your gut health right is so vitally important to your health and weight loss?

Its simple, our gut plays host to approximately 100,000,000,000,000 (100 trillion) microorganisms. To understand how much this is, *"1 million seconds is about 11.5 days, 1 billion seconds is about 32 years while 100 trillion seconds is equal to 32,000 years"*. I hope you can now comprehend how many microorganisms are in our gut.

The human gut contains 10 times more bacteria than all the other human cells in the entire body. There are over 400 *known* diverse bacterial species in our gut. In fact, you could say we are more bacteria than we are human!

We have only recently begun to understand the extent of our gut flora's role in human health and disease. Well, Hippocrates did make this discovery over 2000 years ago but now the medical science world is really taking notice.

Among other things, the gut flora promotes normal gastrointestinal function, provides protection from infection,

17

regulates good metabolism and comprises of over 75% of your immune system. Unfortunately, our modern food production and lifestyle over the past 50-70 years has directly contributed to our unhealthy gut flora. A dysregulated gut flora has been linked to diseases ranging from depression, metabolic syndrome, autoimmune conditions, chronic stress, chronic infections and even autism ASD. Diets high in refined carbohydrates, sugar, processed foods and diets low in fermentable fibres. Dietary toxins like gluten, wheat, industrial seed, soy and oils all directly cause leaky gut.

Also daily intakes of antibiotics and other medications like birth control and NSAIDs *(non-steroidal anti-inflammatory drugs).*

Antibiotics are extremely harmful to our gut flora. Antibiotic side effects cause a profound and rapid loss of diversity and a shift in the composition of our gut flora. In addition, this diversity is ONLY recovered with dietary intervention. We now know that infants who aren't breast-fed and are born to mothers with bad gut flora are more likely to develop unhealthy bacteria in their gut. These early differences in gut flora may predict overweight, diabetes, eczema/psoriasis, depression and other health problems in the future.

## FERMENTED PROBIOTICS VS PROBIOTIC SUPPLEMENTS.

If you look at the shelves of your local health food store, you may be confused by the vast array of probiotic supplements. Probiotics are the buzzword in health these days for a good reason. With benefits ranging from boosting your immunity to easing irritable bowel syndrome, treating autism and ending cravings, it's no wonder we want our probiotics. However, how can you be sure that these probiotics contain all the friendly microflora necessary to build your immunity, help you digest and assimilate your food?

18

# THE BUSINESS OF PROBIOTICS

In a lucrative market, it's no surprise that supplement manufacturers would want a piece of the big probiotic pie. Often, in the race to create a product with so many millions of beneficial bacteria strains and with little to no FDA regulation, one thing is becoming clear: not every supplement manufacturer understands the true nature of healing your inner ecosystem.

So while we know probiotics absolutely have nutritional value, what you see on the label may NOT be what you get.

In fact, two researchers at Bastyr University in Washington recently tested a wide variety of probiotic supplements and found that in four out of twenty products no sign of living friendly bacteria was present.

The unfortunate truth is that too many probiotic supplements vary widely in quality and potency. Here's why, many probiotic supplements cannot survive harsh stomach acid in order to get to your intestines.

Manufacturers talk about number of CFUs (colony forming units), but don't always offer the types or combinations of probiotics that are ideally suited to human intestines. So while they have some value, they do not help re-colonize your inner ecosystem, which is the overall goal.

Just like the Earth has ecosystems that strives for balance, your body has it's own "inner ecosystem." Positioned at the heart of your inner ecosystem are probiotics, the beneficial microflora that keep you healthy, strong and immune from disease and illness. Products containing these beneficial microflora are called probiotics.

19

# BEST PROBIOTICS

Fermented foods and smoothies can be your best solution to ineffective probiotic supplements!

Why are fermented foods and drinks are superior?

Beneficial bacteria and yeast in fermented foods and drinks are alive and active! Whether you buy fermented foods and drinks or make them at home, you are getting real measured *active* bacteria.

Fermentation pre-digests the vital nutrients for you. Packed with B vitamins, minerals and enzymes, fermented foods and drinks are whole foods full of powerful nutritional value in their own right. On top of that, the microflora increase the bioavailability of the nutrients in all the foods you eat by literally hundreds of times.

**Fermentation does not use heat.** Your fermented foods and drinks retain their vital amino acids that are mostly destroyed by heat.

You get a variety of live cultures supplied by nature in fermented foods and drinks. Lab produced probiotics are often a single strain of bacteria, like Lactobacillus acidophilus.

Supplements contain bacteria *only*, while fermented foods and drinks also contain "food" for the microflora to help promote their growth. "It's like sending the good guys down into your digestive tract with a lunchbox of goodies to sustain them on their long and perilous journey. Once they reach their destination (and IF they reach their destination) the microflora in supplement form need up to 6 hours to colonize in your intestines". The microflora in fermented foods and liquids are so hardy they start working at IMMEDIATELY.

Fermented foods and drinks are acid-resistant and are viable in your system from the time they touch your lips all the way down into your gut.

Unfortunately most people have an imbalance between healthy microflora and pathogenic microorganisms, setting the stage for illness and disease. Some of the reasons your inner ecosystem may be imbalanced are:

Antibiotics, recreational or over-the-counter drugs

Too much sugar and other acid-producing foods and drinks.

Environmental toxins

Personal care and cleaning products, including anti-bacterial cleaners.

Poor diet – eating too many processed foods.

Stress, especially chronic stress.

At birth - due to health of the mother prior to or during pregnancy, lack of breast feeding or vaccinations

*So WHAT HAPPENS WHEN YOU START TO CONSUME PROBIOTICS?*

Probiotics are powerful invisible microorganisms that go a long way to turning your digestive and immune health around. In fact in a recent conference at the International Center for Interdisciplinary Studies of Immunology Georgetown University Medical Center, Dr. Michael McCann, MD said:

*"...Probiotics will be to medicine in the twenty-first century as antibiotics and microbiology were in the twentieth century."*

21

## *How much probiotics should you consume? How much is too much?*

Probiotics were once used only for complementary medicine, but they are beginning to get recognition in mainstream medicine today. They are generally thought to be safe and while more studies need to be done, researchers believe you cannot get too much.

You may experience symptoms of "die off," as the "bad guys" (candida, pathogenic bacteria and parasites) die and leave your body. These symptoms can include digestive pain like gas and bloating, headaches, flu-like symptoms and skin eruptions.

Probiotics are an excellent way to create lasting health and as you incorporate them into your diet. Finding a good health care practitioner who can support your natural healing process is a great way to get the support you need. And above all, we are all unique, so listen to your body's signals when trying any new food or supplement.

# OUR GUT BARRIER

Have you ever considered the fact that the contents of the gut are technically outside the body? The gut is a tube that passes from the mouth to your *bum-bum* ☺. Anything that goes in the mouth will pass right out the other end.

This is actually one of the most important functions of the gut to prevent foreign substances from entering your body.

When the intestinal barrier becomes permeable, (leaky gut syndrome) large protein molecules start to escape into the bloodstream. Since these proteins don't belong outside of the gut, the body mounts an immune response and attacks the foreign invaders. Studies have shown that these attacks play a role in the development of autoimmune disease.

In fact, experts in *mucosal biology* now believe leaky gut is a precondition to developing autoimmune disease.

There is also significant growing evidence that increased intestinal permeability plays a pathogenic role in various autoimmune diseases including, celiac disease and type 1-diabetes.

The phrase "leaky gut" used to be confined to the outer fringes of medicine, only employed by alternative practitioners.

Conventional researchers and our Doctors originally refused the idea that a leaky gut contributes to autoimmune problems, now they are seeing the medical evidence is over whelming. It has been repeatedly shown in several well-designed studies that the integrity of the intestinal barrier is a major factor in autoimmune disease.

This new theory holds that the intestinal barrier in large, part determines whether we tolerate or react to toxic substances we

23

ingest from the environment. The breach of the intestinal barrier (which is only possible with a "leaky gut") by food toxins like gluten and chemicals like arsenic or BPA then cause an immune response.

This affects not only the gut itself, but also other organs and tissues. These include the skeletal system, the pancreas, the kidney, the liver and the brain.

This is a crucial point to understand, you really don't have to have gut symptoms to have a leaky gut. Leaky gut can manifest as skin problems like eczema or psoriasis, but can also lead to heart failure, autoimmune conditions affecting the thyroid, Hashimoto's, rheumatoid arthritis, mental illness, ASD (autism spectrum disorder), depression and more.

# INFLAMMATION TRIGGERS THE SYMPTOMS OF DISEASE.

*Inflammation (Latin, īnflammō, "I ignite, Set alight") is part of the complex biological response of vascular tissues to harmful stimuli, such as aspathogens, damaged cells, or irritants.*

The presence of inflammation is what makes most disease noticeable to an individual. It can and often does occur for years before it exists at levels sufficient to be apparent to us or clinically significant. How long it has been present really determines the degree of the severity of a disease and often your prognosis, thus assuming the inflammation can be controlled.

You may now even argue that, without inflammation most disease would not even exist.

Below is listed some of the diseases and their relationship with inflammation.

Before you read on, you need to know what **inflammatory cytokines** are. They are a broad and loose category of small proteins that are important in cell signaling. They are important in health and disease, specifically in their host responses to infection, immune responses, inflammation, trauma, sepsis, cancer, and reproduction.

**Allergies.**

Immune Mediated Types and Sensitivities, all of which cause inflammation.

**Alzheimer's.**

Chronic inflammation destroys brain cells.

25

**Anaemia.**

Inflammatory cytokines attack erythropoietin production.

**Asthma.**

Inflammatory cytokines induce autoimmune reactions against airway lining.

**Autism.**

Inflammatory cytokines induce autoimmune reactions in the brain arresting right hemisphere development.

**Arthritis.**

Inflammatory cytokines destroy joint cartilage and synovial fluid.

**Carpal Tunnel Syndrome.**

Chronic inflammation causes excessive muscle tension shortening tendons in the forearm and wrist compressing the nerves.

**Celiac.**

Chronic immune mediated inflammation damages intestinal lining.

**Crohn's disease.**

Chronic immune mediated inflammation damages intestinal lining.

**Eczema.**

Chronic inflammation of the gut and your liver with poor detoxification.

26

**Fibromyalgia.**

Inflamed connective tissue often food allergy related and exacerbated by secondary nutritional and neurological imbalances.

**Gerd.**

(Gastro esophageal reflux disease), or GERD, is a digestive disorder that affects the lower esophageal sphincter (LES), the ring of muscle between the esophagus and stomach. Symptoms include a burning sensation in your chest / throat and sour taste in your mouth. Chest pain, dry cough or difficulty swallowing. Regurgitation of your food or sour liquid (acid Reflux).

**Kidney failure.**

Inflammatory cytokines restrict circulation and damage nephrons and tubules in the kidneys.

**Lupus.**

Inflammatory cytokines induce an autoimmune attack against connective tissue.

**Multiple Sclerosis.**

Inflammatory cytokines induce autoimmune reactions against myelin.

**Pancreatitis.**

Inflammatory cytokines induce pancreatic cell injury.

**Psoriasis.**

Chronic inflammation of the gut and the liver giving poor detoxification.

27

**Rheumatoid Arthritis.**

Inflammatory cytokines induce autoimmune reactions against joints.

The fact that your immune system drives the inflammatory process in disease is well established in medical research.

Unfortunately, Western medicine offers little in the way of actual answers as to managing or overcoming the autoimmune process. The typical approach to therapy is generally to suppress the immune response with Immune suppressive agents or sometimes steroids.

Both approaches are designed to reduce inflammation but neither stops the underlying disease processes or allows damaged tissues to regenerate.

# WHAT IS A PROBIOTIC CLEANSE?

For many years, I have advocated that a juice detox is by far superior for your health. Juicing provides live nutrients and phytonutrients directly through your liver and into your blood stream. I do however understand that, blending a smoothie provides you all the ingredient fibres, has a slower release rate and therefore a more filling effect when consumed.

I complete a juice detox-cleanse normally every season, (every 3 months) spring, summer, autumn and winter. However I am in constant pursuit for improvement to a healthier way of detoxing, thus providing the complete and maximum effect to your health.

Extensive research over the past two decades has revealed that gut health is now recognized as CRITICAL to our overall health and wellness.

The challenge with a juicing cleanse is you extract the fibre from the juice. However, for an effective probiotic drink we need the fibres to be loaded with probiotics and then digested into the gut. Smoothies are a drink full of fibre, the fibre makes your smoothie way more filling, slow releasing and keeps your hunger satisfied for much longer.

Drinking smoothies with non-probiotic recipes during cleanse can be less beneficial to your gut health. If you want to complete a cleanse, I bet its because you have one of the following symptoms:

- Inflammation,
- Food allergy / intolerance,
- Tired, Fatigued or sluggish,
- Skin allergies
- Suffer insomnia or trouble getting restful sleep.

29

In addition, if you take the birth control pill or if you have recently finished a course of antibiotics then I want to stress this again, medication kills ALL the good bacteria in your gut. When you drink a non pro-biotic smoothie, you consume all of the fibre. The fibres you consume in your smoothie will now sit in your gut as undigested food.

You are now feeding and compounding the bad bacteria in your gut, thus causing more symptoms and inflammation. This in turn causes a vicious cycle of more bad bacteria to develop.

If you only blend prebiotic ingredients, you will achieve a slow recovery detox. Prebiotics feed the good bacteria in your gut. However, these good bacteria need to be present and sufficient in numbers to respond. This can be one of the main reasons for a cleanse failure.

The solution to this problem is to cleanse and detox your body properly and successfully. In order to do so you must start with blending smoothie recipes loaded with fermented probiotics. When you drink these smoothies, the fibres are loaded with probiotics that replenish good bacteria and repair your gut as they are digested.

I have created several delicious recipes that have fermented probiotics that will replenish, repair, strengthen and heal your gut. As you give your body the foundation for good health, you will now focus on power food smoothies that you need while still topping up your healthy bacteria with prebiotics in your smoothies and your raw food.

We then concentrate on hydration, skin care, anti aging, weight loss, Workout recovery, Energy increasing, Heart health, Immunity boosting, Stress beaters, Sex-Mood enhancing, Pregnancy smoothies, Constipation, Healing smoothies, Strong bones and joints, Kid friendly smoothies, Weight loss-Fat burners and much more... (See chapter 7) for 100+ smoothie recipes.

# CHAPTER 2

## SELF-TEST.

## DO I NEED TO CLEANSE / DETOX.

Your symptoms are generally a good indication of whether you have a healthy balance of bacteria in your digestive system. The following is a partial list of common health problems associated with inadequate beneficial bacteria:

A Detoxification self-test is one of the most useful and accurate methods of determining toxin-related health problems. It also serves as a tool for monitoring your health progress. Please answer all questions. If a question does not apply to you, choose never.

**NEVER (0) Rarely (1) Sometimes (2) Often (3)**

**Remember, a score greater than 12 MAY indicate advanced toxin-related health problems.**
Do you drink <u>non</u>-filtered water?

SCORE ___

Do you eat fast foods?

SCORE ___

Do you drink soda?

SCORE ___

Do you drink <u>less than</u> 8 glasses of water a day?

SCORE ___

Do you have <u>less than</u> 2 bowel movements per day?

SCORE ___

Do you suffer bags under your eyes?

SCORE ___

Do you have inflammation or bloating after food?

SCORE ___

Do you have difficulty maintaining / losing weight?

SCORE ___

Do you experience brain fog (difficult concentration or focus)?

SCORE ___

**TOTAL SCORE ___**

**Each of the following are the symptoms of ailments indicating you may need to cleanse and/or change your diet.**

Feeling of being "drained"

Dizziness

Poor Memory Recall

Low Mood / Depression

Lack of energy / Motivation

Irritability

Abdominal Bloating Inflammation

Diarrhea

Sore or dry throat

Loss of sexual desire

Acne or psoriasis

Headaches

Muscle aches

Pain or Swelling in joints

Nasal congestion or discharge

Cough

Belching or intestinal gas

Asthma

Wheezing or shortness of breath.

**How did you score? A score greater than 12** indicates advanced toxin-related health problems and a natural detoxification cleanse is needed.

# DIETS DON'T WORK....EVER !!

Why don't they work?

They always involve a TEMPORARY change in your food and or exercise that resorts back to your normal eating, wait for it.... at the END of your diet. You then end up back to your regular eating plan. What we plan to do here is change a part of your regular diet and slowly increases your consumption of healthy probiotic smoothies, you really wont look back.

We were not predisposed to eat the way we eat today, the book SCOFF NOSH PALEO tell us its only over the past 50 years we have been deceived, or should I say our taste buds have been deceived into eating GMO, parabens, sugar laced pre packaged foods. These foods are all designed to make us get the most out of our day, hence their convenience factor!

The effect of processed food to our health is dramatic, it is now at an epidemic proportion. How many diets and fat free regimes are there? Extreme exercise programs that are good but that are all missing a vital component. REAL balanced continual healthy eating...

It is shown through research that over 95% of people who diet and lose weight gain it back again. The one thing evident is they put themselves and their health under a lot of pressure and stress in doing so.

A gut feeling. Probiotic smoothie diet is designed to retrain your mind, your body *(even your enteric nervous system)* in to eating a healthy diet. More importantly live a healthier, happier life style.

This diet is not about being strict and depriving your body the foods you have been used to eating. This is about being 100% Healthy 80% of the time. YES! Take away the boot camp style

34

pressure and happily change your lifestyle and eating habits gradually, but for GOOD! I guarantee you will prefer the healthy paleo style foods, juices and probiotic smoothies to regular processed foods every time.

So this book will focus on cleansing and detoxing, thus promoting fat loss, then healthy smoothies and recipes to overall improve your health and then your happiness :)

# PROBIOTIC = "FOR LIFE"

# ANTIBIOTIC = "AGAINST LIFE"

# CHAPTER 3

## HEALTH BENEFITS OF EACH FRUIT, VEGGIE & HERB USED IN THE SMOOTHIE RECIPES.

As you read through the following pages you will discover some incredible benefits of fruits, veggies and herbs used in the smoothie diet.

Did you know that every day a fresh fruit sits on the shelf it is loosing essential antioxidants. Freezing your produce the same day, organic fresh picked and frozen produce actually locks in all the essential nutrients for real healthy benefits in your smoothie recipes.

### *PREBIOTIC RICH FRUITS*

Unlike certain vegetables most fruit in its raw state are delicious to eat and easy to incorporate into your daily diet. However, when choosing fruits try and buy fresh organic as much as possible. The older the fruit the faster the vitamins, enzymes and prebiotics degrade. Try and buy only* fresh and organic or fresh picked and frozen organic fruit and vegetables. (See the dirty dozen and the clean 15*).

Fruit can easily be adapted into delicious and healthy dessert dishes such as kiwi fruit mixed with a probiotic yogurt. Another delicious and healthy recipe is a banana smoothie in the morning,

Here is the list of fruits rich in prebiotics

- Apple Skin
- kiwifruit
- Banana
- Cranberries
- Strawberries
- Cherries

## AVOCADO

Has 35% more potassium than bananas. They are rich in vitamin B, E and K. They have high fiber content and help to lower blood cholesterol levels.

## APPLE

Good for your liver and intestines, can relieve diarrhea. Apple skins especially are a great prebiotic, boosting your gut flora and intestinal health.

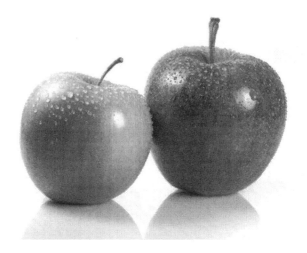

# BANANAS

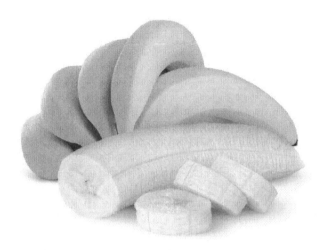

Today, bananas are grown in over 107 countries; they are ranked as number four among the world's food crops for their monetary value. Westerners consume more bananas than ALL the apples and oranges combined.

The banana is the essential base ingredient of your smoothie drink so it is vital to understand the benefits and levels of consumption.

The boasted health benefits of consuming bananas includes lowering the risks of cancer and asthma, lowering your blood pressure, improving your heart health and promoting regularity.

# BANANA NUTRITION

One medium banana (approx. 126 grams) is referred to be one serving of banana.

One serving contains 110 calories, 30 grams of carbohydrate and 1 gram of protein. Bananas are naturally free of fat, cholesterol and sodium. Bananas provide a host of minerals and vitamins including:-

- Vitamin B6 - .5 mg

- Manganese - .3 mg

- Vitamin C - 9 mg

- Potassium - 450 mg

- Dietary Fiber - 3g

- Protein - 1 g

- Magnesium - 34 mg

- Folate - 25.0 mcg

- Riboflavin - .1 mg

- Niacin - .8 mg

- Vitamin A - 81 IU

- Iron - .3 mg

The recommended intake of potassium for adults is 4700 milligrams per day.

# HEALTH BENEFITS OF BANANAS

Eating bananas as part of your regular diet is shown to lower your blood pressure: Also lowering sodium intake is essential to lowering blood pressure, however increasing potassium intake may be just as important because of its vasodilation effect (the widening of blood vessels).

*According to the National Health and Nutrition Examination Survey, fewer than 2% of western adults meet the daily 4700 mg recommended.*

*Bananas have a high potassium intake which is associated with a 20% decreased risk of all inflammation disease.*

**Asthma:** A study conducted by the Imperial College of London found that children who ate just one banana per day had a 34% less chance of developing asthma, impressive!

**Cancer:** Consuming bananas, oranges and orange juice in the first two years of life may reduce the risk of developing childhood leukemia. As a good source of vitamin C, bananas can help combat the formation of free radicals known to cause cancer. High fiber intakes from fruits and vegetables like bananas are associated with a lowered risk of colorectal cancer.

**Heart health:** The fiber, potassium, vitamin C and B6 content in bananas all support heart health. An increase in potassium intake along with a decrease in sodium intake is the most important dietary change that a person can make to reduce their risk of cardiovascular disease, this is according to Mark Houston, MD, Diabetes: Studies have shown that type 1 diabetics who consume high-fiber diets have lower blood glucose levels and type 2 diabetics may have improved blood sugar, lipids and insulin levels. One medium banana provides about 3 grams of fiber.

41

In one study, those who consumed 4069 mg of potassium per day had a 49% lower risk of death from ischemic heart disease compared with those who consumed less potassium (about 1000 mg per day).

High potassium intakes are also associated with a reduced risk of stroke, protection against loss of muscle mass, preservation of bone mineral density and reduction in the formation of kidney stones.

The Dietary Guidelines for Americans recommends 21-25 g per day for women and 30-38 g per day for men.

Treating diarrhea: Bland foods such as applesauce and bananas are recommended for diarrhea treatment. Electrolytes like potassium are lost in large quantities during bouts of diarrhea and may make those affected feel weak. Bananas can help to promote regularity and replenish potassium stores.

Preserving memory and boosting mood: Bananas also contain an amino acid called tryptophan, studies suggest this plays a role in preserving memory and boosting your mood.

Fresh bananas are available all year-round. Most of the smoothie recipes herein use the basis of bananas so get used to buying and freezing them ripe.

Bananas are unlike all other fruits, their ripening process does not slow down after they are picked. Your bananas should normally be stored at room temperature. The warmer the temperature, the faster bananas will ripen. However, you can slow ripen them by chilling them in the refrigerator. Note: the outer peel of the banana will darken but the banana itself will stay intact longer. Adversely to encourage faster ripening, you can place the banana in a brown paper bag at room temperature.

*RISKS AND PRECAUTIONS*

Beta-blockers, a type of medication most commonly prescribed for heart disease, can cause potassium levels to increase in the blood. High potassium foods such as bananas should be consumed in moderation when taking beta-blockers. Consuming too much potassium can be harmful for those whose kidneys are not fully functional. If your kidneys are unable to remove excess potassium from the blood, it could be fatal.

# BLACK BERRIES

These are amazing in smoothies there dark color makes them stand out in fruit salads and desserts, and color your smoothies dark blue, this also indicates their high concentration of antioxidants. Research shows that their vitamin content can help reduce your risk of heart problems, periodontal disease and age-related decline in motor and cognitive function.

Black berries are low in calories, they are virtually fat free, high in fiber and are rich in nutrients, making them an excellent choice for anyone trying to maintain or lose weight in a nutritious manner.

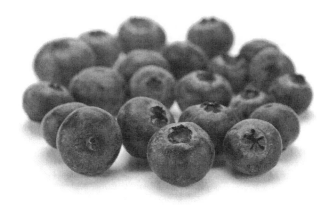

# BLUEBERRIES

Now even more great reasons to enjoy blue berries! This little fruit softens your dry skin, boosts your brainpower, and may even prevent cancer. These help to strengthen your immune system and offer a great detoxifier. Blueberries can even lower your fever.

Berries in general are considered low in terms of their glycemic index (GI). GI is a common way of identifying the potential impact of a food on our blood sugar level once we've consumed and digested that food.

In general, foods with a GI of 50 or below are considered "low" in terms of their glycemic index value. When compared to other berries, blueberries are not particularly low in terms of their GI. Studies show the GI for blueberries as falling somewhere in the range of 40-53, with berries like blackberries, raspberries, and strawberries repeatedly scoring closer to 30 than to 40.

However, a recent study that included blueberries as a low-GI fruit has found that blueberries, along with other berries, clearly have a favorable impact on blood sugar regulation in persons already diagnosed with type 2-diabetes. Participants in the study who consumed at last 3 servings of low-GI fruits per day (including blueberries) saw significant improvement in their regulation of blood sugar over a three-month period of time. (Their blood levels of glycosylated hemoglobin, or HgA1C were used as the standard of measurement in this study.) It's great to see blueberries providing these clear health benefits for blood sugar regulation!

If you want to maximize your antioxidant benefits from blueberries, you gotta go organic! A recent study has directly compared the total antioxidant capacity of organically grown versus non-organically grown high bush blueberries (*Vaccinium corymbosum L.*, var. Bluecrop) and found some very impressive results for the organically grown berries. Organically grown blueberries turned out to have significantly higher concentrations of total phenol antioxidants and total anthocyanin antioxidants than conventionally grown blueberries, as well as significantly higher total antioxidant capacity. Numerous specific antioxidant anthocyanins were measured in the study, including delphinidins, malvidins, and petunidins. The antioxidant flavonoid quercetin was also measured.

# CHERRIES

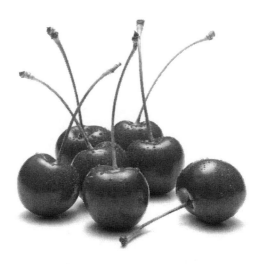

Cherries are a favorite summer fruit. With a short peak season (May to July), high susceptibility to disease and their short shelf life after harvest the cherry season comes and goes, within the blink of an eye.

If you decide to save some for later in the year, put them in your freezer where they will keep for up to one year). Come to September, fresh cherries will be long gone for another year.

## HEALTH BENEFITS OF CHERRIES

Cherries are a member of the same fruit family as peaches, plums, apricots, and almonds, and are often regarded as a "dessert" fruit for use in pies, or perhaps as a garnish for cocktails. Cherries are rich in antioxidants and many other health-promoting compounds.

There are two primary varieties of cherries you should know about: sweet and tart (also known as sour cherries). Sweet cherries, such as Bing cherries, are best eaten fresh (and raw),

46

while sour cherries develop a fuller flavor when they're used in cooking (hence why they're often used for baking).

Tart cherries are also used to make juice concentrates that may offer some unique health benefits. Some of the most notable health effects of cherries include...

Antioxidant Protection

Cherries contain a powerful antioxidant like anthocyanins and cyanidin. One study found the antioxidant activity of these substances isolated from tart cherries was superior to that of vitamin E and comparable to commercially available antioxidant products.

Sweet cherries also contain a small amount of quercetin; this is among the most potent in terms of antioxidant activity and a wide range of other health-promoting properties too.

Cancer-Preventive Compounds

Sweet cherries contain fiber, vitamin C, carotenoids, and anthocyanins, each of which can help to play a role in cancer prevention.

*"The beneficial role of sweet cherries in cancer prevention lies with the anthocyanin content, especially in cyanidin. Sweet cherries are a good source of cyanidins this appears to act as an antioxidant. A study... using human cancer cell lines demonstrated cell cycle arrest and apoptosis of mutated cells exposed to cherry anthocyanins...* ☺

*There is compelling medical scientific evidence that cyanidin may also promote cellular differentiation and thus reduce the risk for healthy cells to transform to cancer."*

Reduce Inflammation

Eating two servings of cherries after an overnight fast lead to a 15 percent reduction in uric acid, and lower nitric oxide and C-reactive protein levels (which are associated with inflammatory diseases including gout).

Consuming tart cherry juice daily for four weeks may lower your levels of uric acid.

Support Healthy Sleep (Melatonin)

Melatonin is a hormone your body produces at night, and one of the primary roles is to help you sleep. But this benefit, for which it is arguably most widely known, is the one of many benefits too!

Additionally did you know melatonin may help protect against heart disease, diabetes, Alzheimer's and migraine headaches? It may also help with weight control and strengthening your immune system? It even appears to play a role in cancer prevention. Cherries contain a natural melatonin, which is a powerful antioxidant and free radical scavenger that helps "cool down" excess inflammation and associated oxidative stress. It also plays a vital role in sleep and bodily regeneration.

Based on daily environmental signals of light and darkness, your pineal gland has evolved to produce and secrete melatonin to help you sleep. Research suggests that consuming tart cherry juice not only help to increase your melatonin levels but may also improve total sleep time and sleep efficiency.

Arthritis Pain Relief

Cherries contain many anti-inflammatory compounds, and research suggests they may help to relieve pain from inflammatory osteoarthritis.

According to one study, women with osteoarthritis who drank tart cherry juice twice daily for three weeks had significant reductions in markers of inflammation. They also had a 20 percent reduction in pain. The researchers noted that tart cherries have the "highest anti-inflammatory content of any food."

Reduce your belly Fat

In an animal study, rats fed tart cherry powder along with a high-fat diet gained less weight and built up less body fat than rats not fed tart cherries. They also had lower levels of inflammation and triglycerides, which is suggested as a potential role in heart health.

Also, athletes who consumed tart cherry juice prior to long-distance running experienced less pain than those who did not. It's thought that the antioxidant and anti-inflammatory properties of tart cherries may have a protective effect to reduce muscle damage and pain during strenuous exercise.

Lowers the risk of stroke

Consuming tart cherries may activate PPAR (peroxisome proliferator activating receptors) in your body's tissues, which help regulate genes involved in fat and glucose metabolism. This activation may help to lower your risk of heart disease, and

49

research suggests eating cherries may provide similar heart benefits to prescription drugs called PPAR agonists Grapes

Also good to purify and strengthen your blood count and good for your colon... Consider fresh organic frozen tart cherries in your diet, so don't overlook these for your smoothies!

# LEMONS

Good for liver and gallbladder, these help with allergies, asthma, cardiovascular disease, and colds.

# ORANGES

Strengthens your immune and nervous system, these are good for cardiovascular disease, obesity, and even varicose veins.

# PEACHES

Improve your skin health, and help to detoxify.

# PEARS

These can help to lower your blood pressure, and are good for your gallbladder.

# PINEAPPLE

Good for your eyes and your skin, and even helps with allergies, arthritis, inflammation and edema.

# STRAWBERRIES

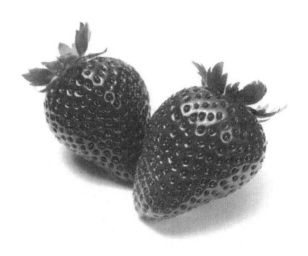

Strawberries are an excellent source of vitamins C and K as well as providing a good dose of fibre, folic acid, manganese and potassium. They also contain significant amounts of phytonutrients and flavonoids which makes strawberries bright red. They have been used throughout history in a medicinal context to help with digestive ailments, teeth whitening and skin irritations. Their fiber and fructose content may help regulate blood sugar levels by slowing digestion and the fiber is thought to have a satiating effect. Leaves can be eaten raw, cooked or used to make tea.

The vibrant red color of strawberries is due to large amounts of anthocyanidin, which also means they contain powerful antioxidants and are thought to protect against inflammation, cancer and heart disease. Great for cleansing the blood, strengthen your nerves and are a strong PREBIOTIC giving a healthy boost to your gut flora and intestinal health.

# HOW TO SELECT AND STORE YOUR STRAWBERRIES

Choose berries that are firm, plump, unblemished and free of mold. Look for those that have a shiny, deep red color and bright green caps attached. Once picked, strawberries do not ripen further so avoid those that are dull, or have green or yellow patches. Wash and handle them with care. Bring to room temperature before serving.

# WATERMELON

Great for your kidneys and also help with edema.

# HEALTH BENEFITS OF VEGETABLE USED IN SMOOTHIES.

Prebiotic fiber is found in many vegetables, such as onions and garlic, ., chicory root

# BEETROOT

This is good for your blood, liver and can help with arthritis and menstrual problems.

# BROCCOLI

One of my FAVORITE vegetables to Juice is broccoli, it is a member of the cabbage family and is closely related to the cauliflower. Originated in Italy. *Broccoli*, means "cabbage sprout".

The health benefits include: -

Detoxification. Broccoli contains a combination of 3 phytonutrients, glucoraphanin, gluconasturtiian, and glucobrassicin. Together these nutrients have a strong impact on your body's detoxification system.

Anti-Inflammatory. Broccoli is a particularly rich source of a flavonoid called kaempferol, which helps in the battle towards allergies and inflammation.

Improves Vitamin D Deficiency. Broccoli contains vitamins A and K, which help to keep the metabolism of vitamin D in balance. Vitamin D promotes the body's absorption of calcium and thereby sustains and promotes bone health, growth and is great for our growing kids.

High in fiber: - Fiber helps to lower cholesterol and facilitates digestion.

Increases eye health. Broccoli improves your eye health due to high concentrations of two carotenoids in it—lutein and zeaxanthin these play an important role in the health of your eyes.

Supports Skin Health And Repair. When glucoraphanin from broccoli is converted into sulforaphane the result is really healthy skin and the repair of any skin damage.

No Wonder we want out kids to eat their greens!

# CABBAGE

Great to ease your colon and even help with ulcers and colitis.

# CAULIFLOWER

Theses are a superfood in their own right and are often widely under appreciated. Cauliflower is a member of the cruciferous family of vegetables. If there is one thing I can stress, it is that cauliflower deserves a regular rotation in your smoothies and your diet. Cauliflower contains a highly impressive array of vitamins, minerals, antioxidants, and other phytochemicals and are rich in choline which can boost your brain health. (See Chapter 4)

# CARROT

There are numerous benefits for your eyes and your skin. Carrots also help you fight infection, helps with arthritis and osteoporosis.

# CELERY

A real strong detoxifier, are great at re-hydrating you and are especially healthy for your kidneys.

# CUCUMBER

Helpful towards dealing with edema and diabetes. Also a great re-hydrator.

# DANDELION

These are great detoxifier and healthy green to add to your smoothie. Dandelion is strong tasting and should only be used with strong flavours to mask the taste.

# JERUSALEM ARTICHOKE

A raw superfood with a delicate, sweet and nutty flavor, Jerusalem artichoke powder can be easily integrated into any daily Smoothie routine. Add the powder to your juices smoothies, baked goods, purées, salads, vinaigrettes, and take pleasure in healthy eating while feeding your beneficial gut flora.

Beyond their prebiotic properties, Jerusalem artichoke is rich in iron, potassium, and vitamin C. Jerusalem artichoke is also a great source of thiamine (B1) and pantothenic acid (B5), a very good source of niacin (B3), as well as a good source of pyridoxine (B6) and riboflavin (B2).

Prebiotic organic Jerusalem artichoke powder contains 65% inulin natural prebiotic. Use in any recipe that calls for a sweetener.

Finally they have one of the highest amounts of prebiotics of most foods Raw Jerusalem artichoke: 31.5% prebiotics by weight They contain small levels of some of the valuable B-complex group of vitamins such as folates, pyridoxine, pantothenic acid, riboflavin, and thiamin.

# LEAFY GREENS

This includes Cabbage, Kale, and Spinach.

A pure detoxifier, good for your skin treats eczema, blood builder and helps with digestion problems and obesity.

# ONION

This helps to lower your blood pressure and also aids your colon.

# POTATOES

These are good for your intestines, also counteracts excess acidity in your stomach.

# RADISH

A Good addition to your smoothies and especially good for your liver cleanse.

# ZUCCHINI

Zucchini is one of the very low calorie vegetables; provide only 17 calories per 100 g. It contains no saturated fats or cholesterol. Its peel is good source of dietary fiber that helps reduce constipation and offers some protection against colon cancers.

Zucchinis have anti-oxidant value (Oxygen radical absorbance capacity- ORAC) of 180 Trolex Equivalents (TE) per 100g, the value is far below some of the berries, and vegetables. Nonetheless, the pods are one of the common vegetables included in weight reduction and cholesterol control programs by most dieticians.

Furthermore, zucchinis, especially golden skin varieties, are rich in flavonoid poly-phenolic antioxidants such as *carotenes, lutein and zea-xanthin.* These compounds help scavenge harmful oxygen-derived free radicals and reactive oxygen species (ROS) from the body that play a role in aging and various disease processes. They are very good source of potassium, an important intra-cellular electrolyte. Potassium is a heart-friendly electrolyte and helps bring the reduction in blood pressure and heart rates by countering the pressure-effects of sodium.

# *W*HAT ARE THE HEALTH BENEFITS OF HERBS?

## GARLIC

Garlic Lowers your blood pressure, fights germs, good for allergies, colds, cardiovascular disease, and diabetes.

## HORSERADISH

Acts as a disinfectant and a diuretic, diuretics are used to treat heart failure liver cirrhosis hypertension and certain kidney disease. Some diuretics, such as acetazolamide helps to make the urine more alkaline free and are helpful in increasing excretion of substances in the cases of overdose or poisoning.

## PARSLEY

A sprig of parsley can provide much more than a decoration on your plate. Parsley contains two types of unusual components that provide unique health benefits. The first type are volatile oil components, the second type is flavonoids.

Parsley's volatile oils myristicin have been shown to inhibit tumour formation in animal studies, and particularly, tumour formation in the lungs. The flavonoids in parsley especially luteolin have been shown to function as antioxidants that combine with highly reactive oxygen-containing molecules (called oxygen radicals) and help prevent oxygen-based damage to cells.

Parsley is also an excellent source of two vital nutrients Vitamin C and Vitamin A (notably through its concentration of the pro-vitamin A carotenoid, beta-carotene).

58

Beta-carotene, another important antioxidant, works in the fat-soluble areas of the body. with beta-carotene-rich foods are also associated with a reduced risk for the development and progression of conditions like atherosclerosis, diabetes, and colon cancer.

Like vitamin C, beta-carotene may also be helpful in reducing the severity of asthma, osteoarthritis, and rheumatoid arthritis. Beta-carotene is converted by the body to vitamin 'a' a nutrient so important to a strong immune system that its nickname is the "anti-infective vitamin."

Parsley is a good source of folic acid, one of the most important B vitamins. While it plays numerous roles in the body, one of its most critical roles in relation to cardiovascular health is its necessary participation in the process through which the body converts homocysteine into benign molecules.

Homocysteine is a potentially dangerous molecule that, at high levels, can directly damage blood vessels. High levels are associated with a significantly increased risk of heart attack and stroke in people with atherosclerosis or diabetic heart disease.

Enjoying foods rich in folic acid, like parsley, is an exceptionally good idea for individuals who either have, or wish to prevent, these diseases. Folic acid is also a critical nutrient for proper cell division and is therefore vitally important for cancer-prevention in two areas of the body that contain rapidly dividing cells—the colon, and in women, the cervix.

The findings, presented in the Annals of the Rheumatic Diseases were drawn from a study of more than 20,000 subjects who kept diaries and were arthritis-free when the study began. Subjects who consumed the lowest amounts of vitamin C-rich foods were more than three times more likely to develop arthritis than those who consumed the highest amounts.

So... next time parsley appears on your plate as a garnish, recognize its true worth and its abilities to improve your health. Also as an added bonus, you'll enjoy parsley's amazing ability to cleanse your palate and your breath at the end of your meal.

# WATERCRESS

A good detoxifier, good for anaemia and helps prevent colds.

# CAYENNE PEPPER

One of the most powerful herbs in the world, with health properties including anti irritant, anti-cold or flu agent, anti-fungal properties helps with migraines, anti-allergen, aids digestion, prevents and treats blood clots, helps sweat during ridding the body of toxins and many other health benefits including a possible anti-cancer agent supports weight loss, lowers appetite, improves heart and blood pressure, helps with gum disease, and is a topical remedy... Just to name a few.

# CINNAMON

Cinnamon (*Cinnamomum velum* or *C. cassia*) has long been considered a "wonder food" in various cultures and science has shown that its active oil components such as cinnamaldehyde, cinnamyl acetate, and cinnamyl alcohol do convey certain health benefits. While the medical research is varied as to the extent of cinnamon's health benefits whether cinnamon can truly combat disease. Cinnamon does have a therapeutic role in certain ailments such as digestive troubles and minor bacterial infections or colds.

While you probably think of it as just a tasty addition to French toast or even rice pudding, the health benefits of cinnamon are numerous. There are many types of cinnamon, but the health

60

studies conducted typically use cassia, the type normally found in grocery stores.

In China, cinnamon has been used for hundreds of years. It is believed to improve vitality, boost energy and increase circulation. It was often given to people who had cold feet, and it is an important ingredient in chai, helping with the digestion of fruits and dairy products.

Other traditional uses for cinnamon include the following: Colds, Nausea, Diarrhea, painful menstruation, Diabetes and indigestion. So start to get creative and sprinkle cinnamon in to some of your own juices, the benefits speak for themselves.

# CORDYCEPS

This is very controversial, this mushroom is believed, by both traditional herbalists and many Western scientists, to be one of the most potent and health improving herbs in the world. Modern science however has very little knowledge about it.

The majority of facts and results have been taken from the studies done by Scientists in China.

It belongs to the family of mushrooms, fungus. The fruiting body of Cordyceps looks like grass. Among the numerous species, Cordyceps sinensis is the most famous due to its curing properties.

The Chinese discovered its powers many centuries ago, having observed that sheep that grazed on Cordyceps were stronger and healthier. Traditional herbalists began using the fungus for curing many diseases in humans. Cordyceps was believed to be a cure-all herb, able to fortify all the body's systems, providing anti-aging, immune boosting, and strength increasing effects.

# SALVIA ROOT

Salvia Root is a traditional Chinese herb that has increasingly become important in the West for supporting cardiovascular health and improving your liver function. It helps to revitalize and detoxify the blood and it is one of the most highly regarded circulatory tonics.

Salvia Root has been shown to inhibit bacterial growth, reduce fevers, diminishes inflammation, ease's skin problems and aid urinary excretion of toxins.

Salvia Root is a member of the multi-species Salvia genus family, and despite the fact that any herb of this genus may be called sage there are significant differences in medicinal components in the tops and roots that influence their uses.

# SPIRULINA.

Spirulina is a natural "algae" (cyanobacteria) a powder that is incredible high in protein and nutrients. When harvested correctly from non-contaminated ponds and water sources, it is one of the most potent nutrient sources available.

It is largely made up of protein 65% (Amino acids and essential amino acids including the essential fatty acid gamma linolenic acid. GLA), and commonly taken by vegetarians for its naturally high iron content.

It is often praised for its high B-12 content, though there is some debate if this particular form is a complete and absorbable form of B-12.

The high concentration of protein and iron also makes it ideal during pregnancy, after surgery or anytime the immune system needs a boost.

# GINGER ROOT

Ginger or ginger root is consumed as a delicacy, medicine or a spice. Preliminary research indicates that there is nine compounds found in ginger that may bind to your serotonin receptors. This may influence gastrointestinal function and promotes the production of bile. Ginger is well known as a remedy for nausea, travel sickness, and indigestion, colic, irritable bowel, loss of appetite, chills, colds, flu, poor circulation, menstrual cramps, dyspepsia (bloating, heartburn, flatulence), indigestion and gastrointestinal problems.

Ginger is a powerful anti-inflammatory herb and there has been much recent interest in its use for joint problems. It has also been recognized for arthritis, fevers, headaches, toothaches, coughs, bronchitis, osteoarthritis, rheumatoid arthritis, to ease tendonitis, lower cholesterol and blood pressure and aid in preventing internal blood clots. Ginger oil has been shown to prevent skin cancer in mice and a study at the University of Michigan demonstrated that gingerols can kill ovarian cancer cells.

## ADD SOME ORGANIC, FERMENTED KEFIR TO YOUR SMOOTHIE.

Kefir contains even more healthy bacteria than yogurt.

To gain the maximum benefit of probiotics try kefir, a creamy, tangy, dairy-based drink that's made when healthy bacteria, mostly lacto bacteria, streptococci, and yeast are introduced into milk. The fermented product is similar in taste to yogurt, except it's a liquid. According to the National Kefir Association, it contains 7 to 10 probiotic cultures, more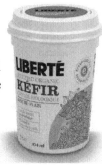

than all yogurts. Kefir is available in the dairy section of most grocery stores, and you can even drink it plain but great used it in your daily smoothie drink. I use liberte' Kefir 454ml tub this is organic fermented cultured bacteria. Kefir is a complex fermented milk product containing bacteria and yeast, it is also recommended by Canada's Food Guide for its calcium content. With over 37 billion bacteria per 100 ml more than any yogurt it's the *champagne* of probiotic milk beverages.

*Kefir does NOT produce symptoms of lactose intolerance, WHY? Because the 37 billion bacteria digest the lactase. Kefir is an excellent source of calcium, potassium, and protein, containing a wider array of digestion-boosting bacteria.*

# MAKE YOUR OWN PROBIOTIC...

Kefir actually means 'feel good" in Turkish. Kefir is an ancient cultured, enzyme-rich food filled with friendly microorganisms. When added to coconut water, Kefir's tart and refreshing flavor is similar to a drinking-style yogurt, and it contains friendly 'probiotic' bacteria. Use with the smoothie recipes adding about one full tablespoon per day to your diet.

To create your very own wonderful fizzy, sour, champagne-like fermented kefir drink teaming with beneficial microflora, simply add a packet of Kefir Starter to coconut water and leave to ferment in a glass preserve jar at a warm room temperature for 36 hours.

It is what it says - a 'starter' meaning you can use it time and again by saving some to start the culture for the next batch. Available on amazon.

# CHAPTER 4

# 9 SMOOTHIE ESSENTIAL SUPER FOODS

## 1. CHIA SEED.

Chia seeds were important to Mayans and Aztecs and they are becoming increasingly popular in modern times. They have been studied for their effects on weight loss, diabetes, and heart health, though results are still preliminary.

Chia means strength, energy booster, chia seed contain healthy omega-3 fatty acids, carbs, protein, antioxidants and calcium. Chia seeds are an unprocessed, whole-grain food that can be absorbed by the body as whole seeds (unlike flaxseeds) however for even easier digestion I recommend ground chia seed. One ounce (about 2 tablespoons) contains 139 calories, 4 grams of protein, 9 grams fat, 12 grams carbohydrates and 11 grams of fiber, plus vitamins and minerals.

The mild, nutty flavor of chia seeds makes them easy to add to foods and smoothies. Chia seeds expand when eaten, helping you to feel full, eat less, and ultimately shed pounds.

## 2. FLAXSEED.

Flaxseed was cultivated in Babylon as early as 3000 BC. In the 8th century, King Charlemagne believed so strongly in the health benefits of flaxseed that he passed laws requiring his subjects to consume it.

Flaxseed is hailed as one of the most powerful plant foods on the planet. There is evidence it may help reduce your risk of heart disease, cancer, stroke and diabetes. These are however quite bold statements for such a tiny seed that's been around for over 13 centuries.

**Omega-3** essential fatty acids, "good" fats that have been shown to have heart-healthy effects. Each tablespoon of ground flaxseed contains about 1.8 grams of plant omega-3s. In studies, the plant omega-3 fatty acid found in flaxseed, called ALA (alpha-linolenic acid), inhibited tumor incidence and tumor growth.

**Lignans,** which have both plant estrogen and antioxidant qualities. Flaxseed contains 75 to 800 times more lignans than other plant foods.

**Fiber**. Flaxseed contains both the soluble and insoluble types.

**Does ground flaxseed have more health benefits than whole flaxseed?**

I recommend ground seed over whole flaxseed, why? Because the ground form of flaxseed is far easier for your body to digest. Whole flaxseed will pass through your intestine undigested, which means you won't get all the benefits of consuming it.

Flaxseed's health benefits come from the fact that they are high in fiber and omega-3 fatty acids, as well as phytochemicals called lignans. One tablespoon of ground flaxseed contains 2 grams of polyunsaturated fatty acids (includes the omega 3s), 2 grams of dietary fiber and 37 calories.

Flaxseed is commonly used to improve digestive health or relieve constipation. They can also help lower your total blood cholesterol and low-density lipoprotein (LDL, or "bad") cholesterol levels, which can help reduce the risk of heart disease.

You can buy flaxseed in bulk, whole or ground at many grocery stores and health food stores. Whole seeds can be ground in a coffee grinder type device and then stored in an airtight container for several months. Refrigerating whole seeds may also extend their freshness.

# CHIA SEED OR FLAXSEED?

All nutritional information is based on **1 ounce (28 grams)** of dried seeds.

**Fibre**: Both of these seeds are a great way to get more fiber in your diet, but chia has the edge: an ounce gives you 10.6 grams of fibre, or 42 per cent of your recommended daily intake, versus 7.6 grams and 31 per cent for flax.

These seeds also provide different types of fibre. Chia is one of the richest sources of soluble fibre, the kind that takes longer to get through your digestive tract, which adds bulk to stool and slows glucose absorption. The fiber in flax, however, is mostly soluble fibre, which has been tied to lower LDL (bad) cholesterol — in fact, research has shown an association between daily flax consumption and lower cholesterol.

**Fat:** Being seeds, both of these are rich in fats. There's a bit more in flax, with 11.8 grams per serving, but chia has 8.6 grams. However, these are healthy fats, including omega 3 fatty acids. A serving of chia has 4915 milligrams of those, while flax has 6388 milligrams.

**Lignans:** Lignans are phytochemicals are linked in reducing cancer risk; in particular, research has suggested that they may have a role in reducing the risk of breast and prostate cancers. Flax is a good source of lignans. Chia seeds also have lignans, but are not as rich a source as flax.

**Protein:** Sprinkling the ground seeds onto your food can up your protein intake. Chia and flax have about the same amount per ounce, at 4.4 grams and 5.1 grams respectively. However, chia is one of just a few plant sources that are a complete protein, meaning, it contains all of the needed protein-forming amino acids. It's not necessary to only eat complete proteins if you get protein in your diet from a variety of sources, but it helps!

**Calcium:** An ounce of flax seeds provides seven per cent of your daily value (DV) of bone-healthy calcium, but chia seeds have more than double: 177 milligrams or 18 per cent of your DV.

**Phosphorus:** Calcium isn't the only mineral that's good for your health — phosphorus is also essential for the formation of bones and teeth. An ounce of flax will give you 180 milligrams of flax or 18 per cent of your recommended daily intake, but chia will give you a whopping 27 per cent with its 265 milligrams of phosphorus.

**Copper:** Copper is a trace mineral important for red blood cell formation, and both chia and flax are good sources. Chia, however, has just a little with three per cent of the recommended daily intake, while flax has 17 per cent.

**How To Eat:** Flaxseeds should be eaten ground as the whole seed is likely to pass through your system undigested, taking all the benefits with it. If you're going to store ground flax, make sure you do so in the fridge in order to prevent oxidation, which will make it taste rancid. Your best bet is to buy flax whole and grind small amounts at a time — a coffee grinder works well for this. Chia seeds, however, can be eaten ground or whole.

**Verdict:** Flax is a seed worth eating, but chia seed has the upper hand thanks to its higher numbers for fibre, calcium, and phosphorus, as well as because it's a complete protein. But all

70

seeds have antioxidants and different kinds, so you should try to get a mix of them in your smoothie diet.

# 3. MACA

Maca has been native to the high Andes of Bolivia and Peru for thousands of years. Maca is actually a herb a member of the cruciferous family of plants. The plant is considered a distant relative of the tuberous root vegetable radish. The Maca plant produces leaves that grow close to the ground and the plant produces a small, off-white flower. Maca root was first observed by German Botanists in 1843, but has been more recently recognized and studied by Peruvian biologists. It grows at an elevation of approximately 10,000-15,000 feet making it probably the highest altitude food-herb crop in the world.

The root grows well but only in cold climates with relatively poor agricultural soils. Although it is mostly cream in color, there are also red and black Maca varieties. The Peruvian cream color is the sweetest in taste and size. Archeological data has shown the predecessors of the Incan people domesticated it over 2,000 years ago. Many indigenous inhabitants of the Andes still view Maca as a valuable commodity.

The Maca root has been used over the ages for its nutritional and herbal qualities. Once harvested, the root was traditionally dried, then ground into powder. Once powdered it was either eaten or put into sacs and traded for other commodities. Maca was also used as money by ancient indigenous peoples. For thousands of years, Maca has been held as a powerful strength and libido enhancer. It is also a powerful adaptogen, which means it has the ability to balance and stabilize the body's cardiovascular, nervous, musculature and lymphatic systems. Impressive.

Maca has the ability to provide more energy if it is needed, but without over-stimulating the body's systems.

Adaptogens also boost your body's immunity and increase the body's overall vitality; this is why the Maca root is so well received today.

According to Peruvian biologist Gloria Chacon de Popivici, Ph.D., Maca alkaloids act on the hypothalamus-pituitary axis and the adrenals. She has theorized that by activating these endocrine glands, Maca is able to increase energy, vitality and libido. In addition Maca improves memory, and blood oxygenation. Maca's actions on sexual function are better researched than its effects on mood and memory.

Maca is dense in nutrition, providing high quality vitamins and minerals. Dried Maca powder is commonly available and contains 60% carbohydrates, 9% fiber, and 10% protein or higher. It has a high lipid profile for a root plant: linoleic acid, palmitic acid, and oleic acid are the roots primary fatty acids.

Maca is rich in minerals containing calcium, magnesium, phosphorous, potassium, sulfur, and iron, and contains trace zinc, iodine, copper, selenium, manganese and silica, as well as vitamins B1, B2, C and E. it actually contains nearly 20 amino acids and seven essential amino acids. Maca is also a rich source of sterols, and is higher in protein and fiber then other root vegetables. Following studies conducted in the U.S., Maca showed absolutely no toxicity and no adverse pharmacological effects. Maca should be used in balance and moderation as with other natural foods. Maca comes in the form of a dried powder and has rapidly gained popularity in the US and in Europe.

It is advised to consume Maca in an organic root powder form. You may use a tablespoon or more of this powder in any natural beverage or food such as smoothies, yogurts, puddings, broths, juices, coffees, homemade chocolates, oatmeal, muffins, cookies and even breads. Maca provides nice flavor to pies and piecrusts. It is also a great emulsifier in foods bringing texture, richness and a very nice consistency. Maca is a powerful super-food and should be consumed in moderation. Up to two tablespoons a day is a good start and, like every herb, I always suggest taking a break from it for a week after about a month of consumption.

# 4. GOJI BERRIES

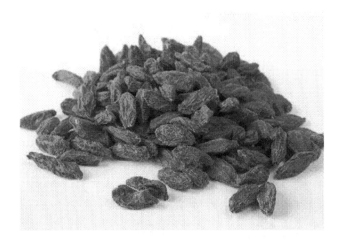

Goji berries (*Lycium barbarum*) are the most nutritionally dense fruit on Earth. They are a member of the nightshade family (*Solonaceae*), which contains many other common vegetables such as potato, tomato, eggplant, and pepper, as well as some poisonous plants like belladonna and deadly nightshade. Native to the Himalayan Mountains of Tibet and Mongolia, the goji berry is now grown in many other countries as well.

Although they have only been introduced in Western countries in recent years goji has been used for thousands of years. It was used in Tibet and China, both as a culinary ingredient and medicine.

Unique among fruits because they contain all essential amino acids, goji berries also have the highest concentration of protein of any fruit. They are also loaded with vitamin C, contain more carotenoids than any other food, have twenty-one trace minerals, and are high in fiber. Boasting 15 times the amount of iron

73

found in spinach, as well as calcium, zinc, selenium and many other important trace minerals, there is no doubt that the humble goji berry is a nutritional powerhouse.

This amazing little super fruit also contains natural anti-inflammatory, anti-bacterial and anti-fungal compounds. Their powerful antioxidant properties and polysaccharides help to boost the immune system. It's no wonder then, that in traditional Chinese medicine they are renowned for increasing strength and longevity.

In traditional Chinese medicine, the goji is said to act on the Kidney and Liver meridians to help with lower back pain, dizziness and eyesight. They are most often consumed raw, made into a tea or extract, or as an ingredient in soups.

Goji are most commonly available in dried form, and make a great snack eaten as is, added to trail mix, muesli or oatmeal. They can also be soaked for a couple of hours in enough water to cover them. Then the soak water can be drained off and makes a delicious drink, or both water and berries added to smoothies.

Please note that there can be adverse interactions if you consume goji berries while also taking medication for diabetes, or blood pressure, or take the blood thinner warfarin. So be sure to consult your health care provider if that is the case.

Goji can often be found in Asian food stores, but most of these come from the commercial growing regions of China and Tibet, and contain high levels of pesticides and synthetic fertilizers. Even some brands that claim to be organic may not be, so be sure to source your goji berries from a reputable source.

# 5. CACAO POWDER

# (HEALTHY RAW CHOCOLATE)

Cacao (ka·cow) is the raw, unprocessed form of chocolate. These untreated seeds called cacao beans can be considered a superfood offering a wealth of antioxidants and essential vitamins and minerals. Is it true that chocolate grows on trees? If you thought "Yes", then you are right.

The superstar of chocolate known as cacao beans are grown on small trees named theobroma cacao, which literally translates to "cacao, the food of the gods" in the Greek language. These trees are native to Mexico, Central and South America. Each cacao pod that emerges from the tree typically houses between 40 and 60 cacao beans. After careful harvesting, the pods are opened, the seeds are removed, and they undergo a natural fermentation and drying process. After the drying process is completed in 1-2 weeks, you are left you with *raw cacao beans*.

To make the chocolate that we all know and love, these raw cacao beans are then roasted to form cocoa, which is then combined with sugar and fats until the beans are unrecognizable. The high heat during the roasting process reduces the levels of antioxidants in the cacao, minimizing the powerful health benefits found in the unprocessed, raw cacao. To receive the greatest benefits from cacao, look for 'raw', non-roasted cacao beans.

Raw Chocolate Health Benefits

Raw chocolate contains many important vitamins and minerals including:

- Magnesium, and other essential minerals including calcium, sulfur, zinc, iron, copper, potassium, and manganese
- Polyphenols called flavonoids, with antioxidant properties
- Vitamins: B1, B2, B3, B5, B9, E
- Essential heart-healthy fat: oleic acid a monounsaturated fat
- Protein
- Fiber

These nutrients found in raw chocolate have been linked to a number of health benefits:

*1) RAW CHOCOLATE CAN LOWER BLOOD PRESSURE &*

*IMPROVE CIRCULATION*

Flavanols, theobromine, and other components found in cacao may lower blood pressure and enhance circulation by promoting dilation, strength, and health of blood vessels

*2) RAW CHOCOLATE CAN PROMOTE CARDIOVASCULAR*

*FUNCTION & HEALTH*

The antioxidant power of flavonoids and essential minerals and vitamins found in cacao can support healthy heart functioning[5] by lowering blood pressure, improving blood flow, lowering LDL cholesterol, and reducing plaque buildup on artery walls.

*3) RAW CHOCOLATE CAN NEUTRALIZE FREE RADICALS*

High levels of antioxidants protect the body from a buildup of free radicals from sun exposure, pollution, cigarette smoking, etc., which may damage healthy body tissue giving rise to cancer and cardiovascular disease.

*4) RAW CHOCOLATE CAN IMPROVE DIGESTION*

A sufficient amount of fiber delivered with each serving of cacao supports digestion while cacao stimulates the body's production of digestive enzymes.

*5) RAW CHOCOLATE CAN ENHANCE PHYSICAL AND MENTAL*

*WELL-BEING*

There are many components of cacao including alkaloids, proteins, beta-carotene, leucine, linoleic, lipase, lysine, and theobromine, that all work together to improve physical and mental health. For example, theobromine helps to stimulate the central nervous system, relax smooth muscles, and dilate blood vessels, giving the body a boost of energy; "bliss" chemicals found in cacao help to increase circulation and availability of serotonin and other neurotransmitters in brain, improving mood and combating depression.

# 6. HEMP PROTEIN

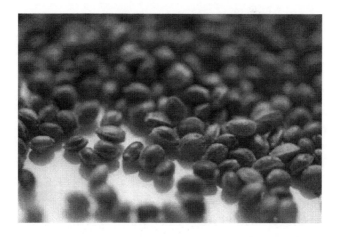

GOOD Hemp proteins are a complete source of protein to support a natural active lifestyle.

Today there are a lot of different protein powders on the market, each have their unique benefits and negatives. However, above all other protein powders, hemp protein has some incredible naturally occurring special properties:

*THE BENEFITS ARE AS FOLLOWS:-*

Hemp is a complete protein.

Hemp is the only protein to contain Omega 3.

Hemp protein is made up of 65% Edestin (The name edestin is from the Greek meaning edible. Hemp protein resembles the globulins found in human blood plasma and is active in DNA repair. Edestin protein sustains life in humans.)

It is easily digested – There is No bloating!

Beneficial PH balance

## WHY IS HEMP PROTEIN SO GOOD?

Hempseed is an excellent source of protein because it contains all the 21 known amino acids. This includes the 9 essential amino acids that the body can't produce on its own and must be taken from dietary sources. Perhaps most vital is the essential fatty acids (Omega-3 and Omega-6); as these do not contain the dioxins and toxins that are common in oily fish (where Omega 3 is also found).

However, unlike soybeans, hemp has not been subjected to genetic modification. While protein is a crucial component for muscle building and repair, so too are vitamins, minerals, fibers, enzymes, probiotics, antioxidants and a host of other nutritional components. However all of these are found in hemp seeds.

Hemp farmers also say that its cultivation hardly requires pesticides, herbicides or petrochemical fertilizers. It happens to be one of those plants that lend easily to organic agricultural methods. This makes hemp a comparatively safer plant source of protein. Two tablespoons of hemp protein powder can provide around 13-15 grams of protein. However it's not just the concentrated quantity that's important here. Those two tablespoons contain what are called branched-chain amino acids (BCAA). Specifically they are leucine, isoleucine, and valine. According to the Food and Agriculture Organization, BCAAs should make up 40% of the daily need for essential amino acids. That breaks down to about 40 milligrams of leucine and 10 -30 milligrams of isoleucine and valine per kilo of body weight.

What's so significant about these amino acids? Along with carbohydrates, they are the fuel that muscles burn for energy. To serve this purpose, their metabolism is more direct and undergoes less processing by the liver, unlike other types of proteins.

It is estimated that up to 18% of energy expended in a workout comes from BCAAs. This can certainly go higher depending on the length and intensity of the exercise. The 40% daily need recommended by the FAO is based on people with regular lifestyles. The figures for daily demand and expenditure during hard physical activities will be higher for athletes.

Use of protein powder is a fairly common practice for athletes as it helps build muscle mass and strength. When choosing a particular powder, you should consider factors such as source and additional nutrients beyond protein. Hemp is a good choice because, as mentioned earlier, it's a safe plant source. The common method of processing hempseeds also allows some of the minerals, vitamins and polyunsaturated fats found in the hull to be mixed in with the ground final product.

**Organic Hemp Protein Powder Practical Uses:**

Hemp protein has a gourmet nutty flavor and is easily blended into a rich, delicious shake.

Protein power shakes are the intended and common preparation for hemp. I have included recipes for pre and post training.

The total nutrients will depend on what else you place in the blender along with the powder. If you want more vitamins and minerals for example, additional fresh fruits would be the best way to go. Some people find hemp protein powder to be bitter. So fruits will improve the taste of your smoothie.

# 7. CAULIFLOWER

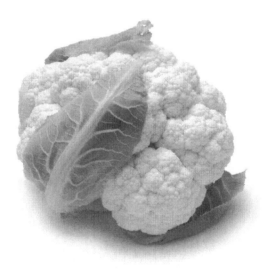

Cauliflower is a member of the cruciferous family of vegetables and is almost overshadowed by its green counterpart broccoli. If there is one thing I can stress, it is that cauliflower deserves a regular rotation in your smoothies and your diet. Cauliflower contains a highly impressive array of vitamins, minerals, antioxidants, and other phytochemicals.

Cauliflower is extremely versatile, raw, added it to salads, and delicious when use it in your smoothies.

It can even be seasoned and mashed for a healthier version of "mashed potatoes." Recently I have used cauliflower for pizza base, hummus and in smoothies making an amazing thick but creamy texture...!!!

Because of its beneficial effects on numerous aspects of our health, cauliflower is what 1 can clearly acknowledge as a superfood. Ten of its most impressive benefits follow:

## 1. Fighting Cancer

Cauliflower contains sulforaphane; this sulfur compound has been shown to kill cancer stem cells, thereby slowing tumor growth. *Some medical researchers believe eliminating cancer stem cells may be the key to controlling cancer.*

Additional research has shown that combining cauliflower with curcumin (the active compound in the spice turmeric) may help prevent and treat prostate cancer.

Health benefits of turmeric include an improved ability to digest fats, reduce bloating, decreases congestion, and improve skin conditions such as eczema, psoriasis, and acne.

A recent study also found sulforaphane inhibits the growth of cultured human breast cancer cells, leading to cell death. Other compounds in cauliflower also show anti-cancer effects according to the National Cancer Institute.

## 2. Boosts Your Heart Health.

Sulforaphane in cauliflower and other cruciferous vegetables has been found to significantly improve your blood pressure and kidney function. Scientists believe the benefits of sulforaphane's are related to improved DNA methylation, which is crucial for normal cellular function and proper gene expression. This is especially crucial in the easily damaged inner lining of the arteries the endothelium.

## 3. Anti-Inflammatory.

It is increasingly common, for the inflammatory response in our bodies to get out of hand. If your immune system mistakenly triggers an inflammatory response when no threat is present, it can lead to significant inflammation-related damage to your body. These conditions are linked to cancer and other diseases, depending on which organs the inflammation is impacting.

Cauliflower contains a wealth of anti-inflammatory nutrients to help keep inflammation in check, including indole-3-carbinol or I3C, (an anti-inflammatory compound that may operate at the genetic level to help prevent the inflammatory responses at its foundational level).

## 4. Rich in Vitamins and Minerals.

Most of the western cultures are seriously lacking in nutrients their body needs to function. Eating cauliflower regularly is a simple way to get these much-needed nutrients into your body. For example, one serving of cauliflower contains 77 % of your recommended daily value of vitamin C. It's also a good source of vitamin K, protein, thiamin, riboflavin, niacin, magnesium, phosphorus, fiber, vitamin B6, folate, pantothenic acid, potassium, and manganese. It is also packed with wrinkle-fighting antioxidants from the sulforaphane's. Impressive ehh?

## 5. Boost Your Brain Health with complete Brain Nutrition.

Cauliflower is a choline rich vegetable, the key ingredient that makes cauliflower such a powerful brain food. Studies show the positive effects of regular consumption of phosphatidylcholine or choline. Studies also show that too little choline may have a negative effect on your brain.

Cauliflower has one of the highest sources of choline, this is a B vitamin known for its role in brain development. Choline is an

82

essential nutrient your body makes in small amounts. However choline must be consumed through the diet for the body to remain healthy. It is used in the synthesis of the constructional components in the body's cell membranes. It also plays a significant role in your nerve communications, prevents the buildup of homocysteine in your blood (elevated levels are linked to heart disease) and reduces chronic inflammation.

In pregnant women, choline plays an equally, if not more, important role, helping to prevent certain birth defects and playing a role in brain development.

**Doubling the RDA of choline during pregnancy protects your baby from stress, metabolic disorders and more...**

Recent research, found the consumption of 930 mg of choline in the third trimester of pregnancy was linked to a 33 percent lower concentration amount of the stress hormone cortisol,. This was compared to those who consumed a RDA of 430 mg.

Babies who are exposed to high levels of cortisol in utero, (such as might occur if a woman is under extreme stress, facing anxiety or suffering from depression), have an increased risk of stress-related and metabolic disorders. The research indicates the beneficial impact of choline on lowering cortisol can actually protect the baby later in life from mental health conditions, high blood pressure and type 2 diabetes.

Interestingly, the higher choline intake led to changes in epigenetic markers in the fetus. Specifically, it affected markers that regulate the hypothalamic-pituitary-adrenal (HPA) axis, this controls hormone production and activity. The higher intake of choline contributed to a more stable HPA axis, which in turn meant lower cortisol levels in the fetus. The changes in fetal genetic expression will likely continue into adulthood, where they play a role in disease prevention.

### 6. Detoxification Support

Cauliflower helps your body's ability to detoxify in a multiple of ways. Cauliflower contains antioxidants that support Phase 1 detoxification along with sulfur-containing nutrients important for Phase 2 detox activities. The glucosinolate in cauliflower also activate our detoxification enzymes

### 7. Digestive, Prebiotic Benefits

Cauliflower is an important source of dietary fiber for digestive health. "Researchers have determined that the sulforaphane made from a glucosinolate in cauliflower (glucoraphanin) can help protect the lining of your stomach. Sulforaphane provides you with this health benefit by preventing bacterial overgrowth of Helicobacter pylori in your stomach".

### 8. Antioxidants and Phytonutrients

Eating cauliflower is akin to winning the antioxidant and phytonutrient lottery. Yes Cauliflower is packed with vitamin C, beta-carotene, kaempferol, quercetin, rutin, cinnamic acid, and much more. Antioxidants are nature's way of providing your cells with adequate defense against attack.

# 8. AVOCADO.

Apart from being a very good source of fiber and vitamins, research shows there are a number of other benefits associated with the fruit, including:

Lowering cholesterol levels,

Reducing the risk of diabetes,

Promoting lower body weight,

Preventing cancer.

Avocados cab also help to lower cholesterol

Researchers suggest that eating avocados could help lower levels of bad cholesterol. A study published in the Archives of Medical Research found that an "avocado enriched diet can improve lipid profile in healthy and especially in mild hypercholesterolemia suffering patients.

After a week of following the avocado enriched diet the patients experienced a 22% decrease in bad cholesterol and triglyceride levels and an 11% increase in good cholesterol. Avocados may also reduce the risk of diabetes, stroke, and coronary artery disease

Metabolic syndrome (The group of symptoms that increase the risk of diabetes, stroke, and coronary artery disease). One study, published in a Nutrition Journal assessed the link between avocado consumption and metabolic syndrome. The scientists concluded, "Avocado consumption is associated with improved overall diet quality, nutrient intake, and reduced risk of metabolic syndrome."

Avocados may promote a healthy body weight and BMI. The same study (as the one referenced above), titled "Avocado consumption is associated with better diet quality and nutrient intake, and lower metabolic syndrome risk in US adults", also found that people who ate avocados were more likely to have a lower body weight, BMI (body mass index), and waist circumference.

Avocados may also help to prevent cancer.

Avocados are rich in phytochemicals, which have been reported to help prevent the development of certain cancers. A team of scientists who examined the chemo preventive characteristics of avocados concluded, "individual and combinations of

85

phytochemicals from the avocado fruit may offer an advantageous dietary strategy in cancer prevention."

# RISKS AND PRECAUTIONS

Although this is very rare, avocado allergies do exist. According to a case report published in the journal *Allergy, Asthma & Clinical Immunology*, avocado allergies are associated with "coughing, wheezing, nasal stuffiness, generalized urticarial and periorbital edema."

# 9. SPINACH

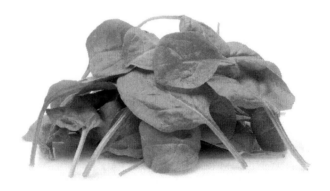

I think Popeye was definitely on to something here! Spinach is a real super food loaded with tons of nutrients in a low calorie package. All dark leafy greens like spinach are important for skin and hair, bone health, and provide protein, iron, vitamins and minerals.

The health benefits of consuming spinach include improving blood glucose control in diabetics, lowering the risk of cancer, lowering blood pressure, improving bone health, lowering the risk of developing asthma and more.

**As with all these super foods it is important to consult your doctor if you begin to experience any unpleasant side effects after adding them to your diet.**

CLEANSE-HEAL-ENERGISE & LOSE WEIGHT

# CHAPTER 5

# THE MIRACLE WATER CURE

## LET US COVER YOUR WATER INTAKE.

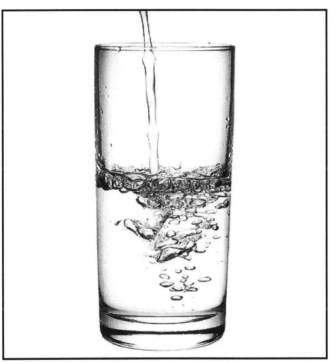

**Statement:** 80% of us are chronically dehydrated, we mistake our thirst for hunger and we tend to eat when our bodies are trying to tell us we are in fact thirsty and just need hydrated.

Yes most of us know this already…right? But how many of us can honestly say we follow the guidelines for keeping us properly hydrated?

# THE HEALTH BENEFITS OF WATER.

Did you know that water is the body's main chemical compound and makes up a whopping 60% of your total body weight? All the systems in your body depend on water to maintain health. Water flushes out toxins from your vital organs. Water carries nutrients to our cells and provides a moist environment for our ear, nose and throat tissue.

A lack of water can lead us to dehydration and chronic health issues. Even without this juicing diet I urge you, if you want to vastly improve your health drink your daily-recommended water intake.

# HOW MUCH WATER SHOULD I DRINK?

You lose water from your body through your breath, perspiration, urine and bowl movements. For your body to function properly we must replenish our water supply by consuming water and foods that contain water every day.

# THE INSTITUTE OF MEDICINE RECOMMENDS:

Men: 3.0 liters or 10 cups a day.

Women: 2.2 liters or 6-7 cups a day.

Pregnant women 2.4 liters or 7 cups a day.

Breast-feeding women: 3.0 liters or 10 cups a day.

Exercise: add an extra 2 to 3 cups a day.

Environment: hot / humid weather or heated air increase your water intake.

Higher altitudes: Increased urination and breathing increase your water intake.

Sickness: vomiting, diarrhea, bladder infections and urinary tract stones should also increase your water intake.

***Please note: -***

*1 - cup of water is on average measuring 1/3 liter or 333 ml. 1 tall glass of water is on average measuring 425 ml.*

Water aides in flushing toxins out of the body and improves detox cleanse effectiveness.

CLEANSE-HEAL-ENERGISE & LOSE WEIGHT

# CHAPTER 6

## NOW LETS START THE 3-10 DAY

## SMOOTHIE CLEANSE.

Follow this cleanse using the recipes and you will find a major benefit if you have any of the symptoms mentioned throughout chapter 1.

Complete this cleanse following the 3-10 day recipe plan. Use the kefir probiotics supplement directly in every morning smoothie. This is your full RDA of probiotics. Remember you are consuming prebiotics throughout your cleanse. Consuming prebiotics can actually double your good bacteria in as little as 2 hours after drinking.

This cleanse is not about starving yourself, in fact its an over indulgence of phytonutrients, vitamins and minerals.

During the cleanse drink 3 large smoothies Breakfast, mid morning / afternoon, lunch. Then eat one healthy meal per day for dinner.

**Drink filtered water.** Remember these smoothies are NOT supplements they are a meal. During your cleanse you <u>must</u> drink your RDA of water. This will not only rehydrate you but will help with flushing the toxins out of your body.

**Try to buy organic.** See the dirty dozen and the clean 15 in chapter 8.

**Only consume nutrient rich foods** and snacks high in minerals, vitamins, fiber and omega 3 fatty acids. NO JUNK FOODS, these contain empty calories, and are loaded with sugars. You want all your calories to provide you with nutritional values that will help to heal your body and maintain a healthy weight.

**Avoid ALL wheat, gluten, sugar**, trans fats and salt. Do not eat processed foods, cereals or breads.

**Eat at least 30 grams of fiber per day**, studies show this high fiber diet protects you against cancer, stroke, heart disease and also helps you to loose weight.

**Eat proteins, white meats,** chicken, pork, nuts or fish and limit your red meat intake to maximum 2 times per week. Red meats contain alot of saturated fats. White meats contain the essential fats your body needs.

**Eat 4 if not 5 times a day,** (3 meals and 2 healthy snacks) this will help you loose more weight quickly. When you eat this way (eat every 3 to 4 hours, you are stimulating your metabolism in shorter bursts, therefore the more often you eat the faster your metabolism is.

Each 1-10 day recipe is enough to make 3 large healthy smoothie drinks / remember these are full MEALS.

After your cleanse you must drink at least one smoothie per day, preferably in the morning, getting all the nutritional value into your body every single day. When you find your favourite recipes add one of the super foods we've covered in chapter 4.

Rotate your greens and vary them every week. All greens have alkaloids in them. By rotating your greens, you prevent any chance of alkaloid build-up and you expose yourself to a variety of nutrients found in these wonderful foods. Plus, each leafy green provides different phytochemicals, vitamins, minerals, micro- and macronutrients and antioxidants.

Your body needs these to perform at its best. Some alkaloids found in nature have been shown to provide health-promoting

94

properties, like the ability to boost immunity, promote heart and muscle-calming effects, house anti-asthma therapeutic properties, and help lower elevated blood sugar.

# LETS GET STARTED.

The night before starting your 3-10 day Smoothie Cleanse it is advised that you take a laxative herbal tea.

The first morning and each morning following, you should take a lukewarm glass of purified / filtered water with one teaspoon of <u>uniodized sea salt</u>. The salt water is absorbed quickly in to your bloodstream and helps to flush out the toxins in your digestive tract.

The herbal tea also helps alongside the salt water to rid the waste from the body. Alternatively a fresh squeezed lemon juice and water drink can replace this <u>after</u> the first day.

Between the saltwater mixture and the nightly herbal laxative tea you are to consume 3-4 glasses of the Smoothie meal full of anti-oxidants fibre and protein per day.

You may also occasionally drink green tea or peppermint tea with no sugar added as your daily treat.

It is advised that the Smoothie mixture is made up in larger containers that helps bulk servings and prevents you from tiring of individual servings. I use the Ninja Pro blender with a 2.15 Ltr blending capacity, (about 9 cups / 2150 ml) this is more than sufficient to blend my full 3 single serve smoothie meals in one prep. These can keep refrigerated for up to 1-2 days with a sealed lid too!

An important part of your cleanse is to rest, drink 2-4 glasses of purified filtered water daily. You can take a low to moderate rate of exercise like walking the dog, faster pace walking, taking the stairs at work, or even a low intensity exercise class.

Its 3-10 days, so know your limits…

## AN EXAMPLE OF A TYPICAL DAY OF THE CLEANSE DIET.

**3-4 Smoothie cleanse drinks per day.**

**2-4 glasses of purified filtered water per day** (see RDA Chapter 5).

## MORNING. (FIRST THING)

Flush with the saltwater mixture or 1 glass of water and fresh lemon juice and one drink of purified filtered water.

*Once your happy with your smoothies please feel free to mix it up a bit and take advantage of the different smoothies giving you a host of different benefits.*

## BREAKFAST.

One drink of purified filtered water. Day one nutritional Smoothie drink to get you started. You could even try the **Strawberry, Banana & Grape Smoothie** ⊕ this smoothie gives your energy levels a boost, awakens your digestive system while giving your body nutrition.

If you are keen to get your '5-a-Day' this is an excellent start for your cleanse!

# LUNCH.

Drink one glass of purified / filtered water. One nutritional Smoothie as you progress and become comfortable with the smoothie recipes try and target different areas of your body, i.e. if your immune system is low, you suffer from digestion problems or you have high cholesterol then choose the recipe that benefits you.

# MID AFTERNOON

Drink one glasses of purified / filtered water. Then drink your final days smoothie.

# DINNER.

A great one can be the soup recipe that includes the broccoli soup. Chicken salad, Fish and greens steamed.

There are so many good recipes. I can send you a copy of my Paleo book Scoff Nosh Paleo just email me at olivermichaels.author@hotmail.com. This book has an abundance of easy healthy recipes.

**Once you're at the end of your first detox diet here are some suggestions you can adopt into your everyday life and diet: -**

* Drink at least one Smoothie a day; this can be a cleansing Smoothie or energy breakfast drink.

* Lightly steam all your vegetables allowing it to lock in and retain all the nutrients and great taste.

* Increase the consumption of organic foods where you can, if you have space, why not set up a raised garden and grow a lot of your own vegetables? At least you will know where your produce is coming from and know it's organic.

* Use herbs on your everyday foods like the amazing cayenne pepper, sprinkled over white / red meats or fish, you can also add cordyceps, parsley, ginger root and salvia root to your foods and juicing drinks too.

* Keep your body hydrated, drink purified filtered water. Did you know about 80% of people are dehydrated? Your body can't determine hunger between thirst and you generally turn to food when in fact you just need re hydrated.

* Every three months whilst maintaining the healthy detox diet, complete the detox cleanse diet for your whole body.

* Every three months while maintaining the healthy detox diet, complete the 3-10 day Smoothie cleanse diet.

**EACH OF THE FOLLOWING 1 TO 10 DAYS RECIPES PROVIDES YOU 3 SMOOTHIE DRINKS FOR YOUR FULL DAYS CLEANSE.**

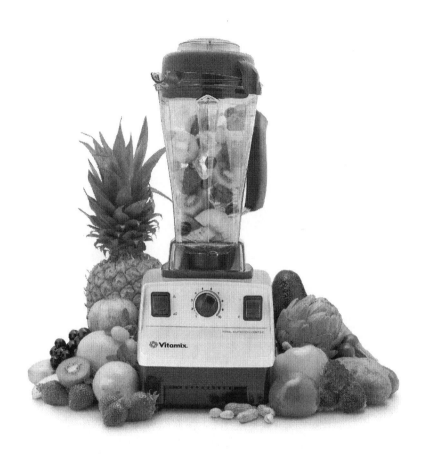

# DAY 1

**The Very Berry Green Smoothie**

**Number of Ingredients – 8/9**

**Time to prepare 6 min**

1 tablespoon Kefir - fermented probiotic

3 handfuls of fresh spinach or other greens

2 cups of water

1 apple cored, and quartered

1 - cup frozen strawberries

1 handful of frozen seedless grapes

1 - cup frozen mango (optional)

1 packet stevia (optional)

2 tablespoons of ground chia seed

*Optional 1 scoop of protein powder.

Blend adding your required fluid amount until creamy and enjoy, keep refrigerated and consume throughout the day.

# DAY 2

**The Very Berry Green Smoothie**

**Number of Ingredients – 7/8**

**Time to prepare 5 min**

**Apple, Banana & Strawberry Smoothie**

1 tablespoon Kefir - fermented probiotic

3 handfuls of fresh spinach or other greens

2 cups of water

1 large banana, peeled

2 apples, cored, and quartered

2 cups frozen strawberries

2 packets of stevia (optional)

2 tablespoons ground Chia seed

Place the greens and water into your blender and blend until mixed fully. Now add the remaining ingredients and blend until creamy and delicious.

# DAY 3

### The Very Blue Apple Berry Smoothie

### Number of Ingredients – 9

### Time to prepare 5 min

### Blue Apple & Berry Smoothie

1 tablespoon Kefir - fermented probiotic

1 handful broccoli stems and 2 handfuls spinach

2 cups of water

11/2 cups of frozen blueberries

1 banana, peeled

1 apple cored and quartered

1 packet of stevia

2 tablespoons ground flax seed

Optional 1 - cup of protein powder

Place the greens and water into your blender and blend until mixed fully. Now add the remaining ingredients and blend until creamy and delicious.

# DAY 4

**The Very Peachy Berry Smoothie**

**Number of Ingredients – 9**

**Time to prepare 5 min**

1 tablespoon Kefir - fermented probiotic

2 handfuls of kale and 1 handful spinach

2 cups water / almond milk

2 apples, cored, quartered

1 1/2 cups frozen peaches

1 1/2 cups of frozen mixed berries

2 packets of stevia

2 tablespoons ground flax seed

Optional 1 - cup of protein powder

Its day 4 and now were really on the way to enjoying healthy food. Place the greens and water into your blender and blend until the mixture is green-like consistency. Add remaining ingredients. Blend until rich, creamy and delicious.

# DAY 5

**The Berry, Peach & Spinach Smoothie**

**Number of Ingredients – 7**

**Time to prepare 5 min**

**Blue Apple & Berry Smoothie**

1 tablespoon Kefir fermented probiotic

3 handfuls of Spinach

2 cups water

1 - cup of frozen peaches

1 handful fresh or frozen seedless grapes

11/2 cup of blueberries

3 packets stevia to sweeten

2 tablespoons ground flax seed

Optional 1 - cup of protein powder

Place the greens and water into your blender and blend until the mixture is green-like consistency. Add remaining ingredients. Blend until rich, creamy and delicious.

# DAY 6

**The Pineapple Spinach Smoothie**

**Number of Ingredients  – 7/8**

**Time to prepare 7 min**

**Blue Apple & Berry Smoothie**

1 tablespoon Kefir fermented probiotic

2 cups of fresh spinach packed

1 - cup of pineapple chunks

2 cups frozen peaches

2 bananas, peeled

1-2 packets stevia

2 cups water

Optional 1 - cup of protein powder

Place the greens and water into your blender and blend until mixed fully. Now add the remaining ingredients and blend until creamy and delicious.

# DAY 7

### The Pineapple & Berry Smoothie

### Number of Ingredients – 10/11

### Time to prepare 6 min

1 tablespoon Kefir fermented probiotic

2 handfuls spring mix greens

2 handfuls of spinach

1 banana, peeled

11/2 cups of pineapple chunks

11/2 cups frozen mango chunks

1 - cup frozen mixed berries

3 packets of stevia

2 cups of water

2 tablespoons of ground flax seed

Optional 1 - cup of protein powder

Place the greens and water into your blender until mixed fully. Now add the remaining ingredients and blend until creamy and delicious.

# DAY 8

**The Spinach Kale Berry Smoothie**

**Number of Ingredients – 9**

**Time to prepare 6 min**

1 tablespoon Kefir fermented probiotic

2 handfuls kale

2 handfuls of spinach

2 cups of water

1 apple, cored, quartered

1 banana, peeled

11/2 cups frozen blueberries

2 packets of stevia

2 tables spoons ground flaxseeds

Optional 1 - cup of protein powder

Place the greens and water into your blender until mixed fully. Now add the remaining ingredients and blend until creamy and delicious.

# DAY 9

### The Mango and Apple Smoothie

### Number of Ingredients – 9

### Time to prepare 6 min

1 tablespoon Kefir fermented probiotic

3 handfuls spinach

2 cups water

1 apple, cored, quartered

11/2 cups mangoes

2 cups frozen strawberries

1 packet of stevia optional

2 tablespoons ground flaxseeds

Optional 1 - cup of protein powder

Place the greens and water into your blender until mixed fully. Now add the remaining ingredients and blend until creamy and delicious.

# Day 10

**The Peach and Pineapple Kale Smoothie**

**Number of Ingredients – 9**

**Time to prepare 5 min**

1 tablespoon Kefir fermented probiotic

2 handfuls kale

1 handful spring mixed greens

2 cups water

11/2 cups frozen peaches

2 handfuls pineapple chunks

2 packets of stevia

2 tablespoons ground flaxseeds

Optional 1 - cup of protein powder

Place the greens and water into your blender until mixed fully. Now add the remaining ingredients and blend until creamy and delicious.

# CHAPTER 7

## 101 SMOOTHIE RECIPES FOR HEALTH AND VITALITY.

With all the following recipes you can add 1 tablespoon Kefir fermented probiotic to re establish your gut health. Recipes marked ⊕ are recipes high in prebiotics, fruits and vegetables that will feed the good bacteria already present. Feel free to change and design your own recipes. You will no doubt find your favourite mixes. The recipes are listed in the healing and health-benefiting category. Enjoy your smoothies!

## DETOXIFICATION

**Blackberry & Banana Smoothie** ⊕

2 handfuls greens

¼ cup water

1 banana, peeled frozen

½ cup frozen blackberries

1 - cup frozen strawberries

1 - cup frozen blueberries

2 handfuls greens

1-cup water

**Apple Banana Smoothie** ⊕

2 handfuls green

1 - cup ice

2 granny smith apples, cored and seeded

2 small bananas, peeled

## Mango & Pineapple Smoothie

2 handfuls greens

11/2 cups coconut water

1 - cup frozen mango chunks

1 lime, peeled and seeded

Pinch cayenne pepper

## Pear & Pineapple Smoothie

2 handfuls greens

1 - cup ice

1 pear, seeded

1 small apple, cored and seeded

2 cups pineapple chunks

## Grapefruit & Banana Smoothie ⊕

2 handfuls greens

1-cup water

1 banana, peeled and frozen

1 - cup frozen strawberries

1 pink grapefruit, peeled and seeded

1 packet stevia.

**Lemon & Lime Smoothie**

2 handfuls greens

1 large fresh- squeezed orange

½ cup ice

2 bananas, peeled and frozen

½ lemon, peeled and seeded

½ lime, peeled and seeded

# DIABETES/BLOOD SUGAR CONTROL

**Orange & Plum Smoothie**

2 handfuls greens

1/2-cup ice

2 oranges peeled

½ cup plums

113

1-teaspoon cinnamon

2 tablespoons of flaxseed

**Pear & Banana Smoothie**

2 handfuls greens

1 - cup almond milk

1 banana, peeled and frozen

1 pear cored and seeded

1 apple cored and seeded

1 teaspoon of cinnamon

**Kiwi & Almond Smoothie** ⊕

2 handfuls greens

11/2 cups almond milk

1 banana, peeled and frozen

2 kiwis (skin on)

1 - cup frozen strawberries

2 tablespoons ground flaxseeds

**Berry & Banana Smoothie**

2 handfuls greens

1-cup water

1 banana, peeled and frozen

11/2 cups frozen berries

2 tablespoons of flaxseed

**Mango & Almond Smoothie**

2 handfuls greens

11/2 cups almond milk

½ cup frozen mango chunks

1 - cup frozen strawberries

**Mango & Orange Smoothie**

2 handfuls greens

1-cup water

½ cup frozen mango chunks

½ lemon, peeled and seeded

1 orange, peeled and seeded

2 tablespoons sunflower seeds

115

## Avocado & Greens Smoothie ⊕

2 handfuls greens

1-cup water

1 Med banana, peeled

2 cups frozen strawberries

¼ avocado, peeled


## Orange & Berry Smoothie

2 handfuls greens

1 - cup unsweetened almond milk

1 small orange peeled

½ cup mixed berries

1 teaspoon goji berries, soaked for 10 minutes (powdered goji has better absorption into the body)

1 tablespoon of ground flaxseed

1 scoop of Hemp protein alternative

# ENERGY / PRE WORKOUT SMOOTHIES INFO

There are some advantages to knowing how your body works and what it needs to perform at its best. The bottom line for healthy weight loss and fitness sounds simple: you have to eat fewer calories than you use up but not fewer than your body needs to function at its best.

The size, timing, and content of your pre- and post-exercise meals and snacks can play an important role in your energy levels during your workout, how well your body recovers and rebuilds after your workout, and whether the calories you eat will be used as fuel or stored as fat. Here's what you need to eat and drink to get the results you want!

## YOU NEED PRE-EXERCISE FLUID

Being well hydrated will make your exercise easier and more effective. Try to drink 16-20 ounces of water during the 1-2 hours before starting your workout.

## YOUR PRE-EXERCISE MEAL OR SNACK

News flash: Most of the fuel you use during exercise doesn't come from the food you've recently eaten! It actually comes from the carbohydrates (called "glycogen") and fat that's stored in your muscles, liver, and fat cells. That's enough to fuel 1-2 hours of very intense exercise or 3-4 hours of moderate intensity exercise.

This means that if your overall diet is adequate to keep your fuel tanks topped off, you may not need to eat anything before you work out. So, if eating before exercise upsets your stomach or you like to exercise first thing in the morning or at a time when eating first isn't convenient, don't feel like eating first is a must.

Some people do have a hard time exercising without eating first, especially if it's been a long time since their last meal or snack. These individuals often are more sensitive to changes in their blood sugar levels, which fall during the first 15-20 minutes of workout. That drop in blood sugar can cause tiredness, mild dizziness, or even faintness—especially if your blood sugar was already low, but eating something beforehand can help prevent this.

If you have health issues like diabetes or hypoglycemia that can cause low blood sugar, you'll probably want to eat before your workout. If you get very hungry during a workout (and it interferes with your energy levels or focus), or become so ravenous after an exercise session that you end up overeating, try eating before you hit the gym to avoid these problems.

If you are a moderate exerciser who tends to perform better with a pre-exercise snack, there are two ways to handle your needs:

1. Eat a small (100- to 200-calorie) snack about 30 minutes before you work out. This snack should include fast-digesting (high glycemic index) carbohydrates and very little fat (which digests slowly), so that you digest the meal quickly and the fuel is available during your exercise session. Here are some ideas:

- Fruit juice /Smoothie

- High-glycemic fruits like pineapple, apricots, banana, mango, and watermelon

**2. Eat a nutritionally balanced meal 1-2 hours before your exercise.** This is the best option for many people. The larger the meal, and the more fat and protein it contains, the longer you may need to wait before exercising. Ideally, try to eat enough calories to equal about half the calories you expect to burn during your upcoming workout.

So if you burn about 600 calories during your workout, aim for at least 300 calories during this meal — or a little more if your exercise is "high intensity" (over 75% of your maximum heart rate). At least 50-60% of these calories should come from carbohydrates, which should keep your blood sugar and energy levels fairly stable during your exercise session.

Include some protein to help prevent the breakdown of muscle for fuel and give your muscles a head start on recovery after exercise. Some good food choices and combinations for this kind of meal include:

- Fruit and kefir probiotic

- Nuts

- Trail mix with nuts and dried fruit

- Hummus and raw veggies

- Hard boiled eggs (or egg whites)

- Cottage cheese and fruit

- Half a peanut butter or turkey/chicken

- Tomato or vegetable juice

- Smoothie (with added protein powder, if desired)

## Question; Should I drink my protein shake pre- or post-workout?

You can take in protein or amino acids pre- and post-workout, but following all my research and if I absolutely had to pick, I would say pre-workout. Yes! before the workout, and here's the reason why…

Post workout shakes have long been considered as the most important piece of the workout nutrition puzzle. However, the most recent research suggests that ingesting your protein and amino acids prior to training can be even more beneficial for you.

Pre-workout protein, specifically the branch chain amino acids (BCAAs), will help to fuel your muscles during training. Because BCAAs don't need to be processed by your liver after being absorbed, they can head directly into your blood stream to be used up by your muscles.

This is actually key as exercise causes the breakdown and oxidation of BCAAs. Providing BCAAs to working muscles will prevent the need for your body to catabolize (breaks down) the working muscle itself. So adding protein prior to your training session primes the pump: It starts protein synthesis during rather than after your training session, which in turn causes increased Protein Synthesis.

Pre-workout protein will likely increases amino acid delivery and uptake by muscles during training. Taken alone or as part of a complete protein, BCAAs inhibit muscle breakdown. So the net protein synthesis is elevated even higher!

Burn More Calories

A recent study published in Medicine and Science in Sports & Exercise found that one scoop of *whey protein* prior to working out increased calorie burning over the subsequent 24 hours. *I know we are using natural organic hemp protein with this, there are even greater benefits to you.*

The exact cause of this increase in calorie burning is unknown, but it may be due to the added metabolic effects of increasing protein and modifying substrates (energy sources) that are used during your exercise.

But please don't wait for the boffins and the eggheads: Why not reap the benefits of the (increased calorie burning!) without knowing the exact scientific metabolic cause why.

120

There is also a carryover effect of nutrients taken in the pre-workout period. After ingesting protein, muscle protein synthesis can stay elevated for as long as up to 3 hours.

So this actually means that your pre-workout protein smoothie allows you to double dip: You will reap the benefits of elevated blood amino acids during your training session in addition to a carryover of elevated blood amino acid levels after your workout too.

This elevation of blood amino acids will also help prevent excessive post-workout muscle breakdown.

This occurs partly through the reduction of the muscle-catabolizing hormone cortisol. A 2007 study published in the Journal of Strength and Conditioning Research found that starting your workout nutrition with a protein-and-carbohydrate shake 30 minutes prior to exercise led to a significant reduction in cortisol up to one day following the training session.

Fat-Burning Bonus

Taking protein (specifically BCAAs) alone before a workout is extremely beneficial during a low-carb diet. The consumption of pre-workout BCAAs, especially when glycogen levels are low (as they are during a low-carb diet), leads to an increase in fat oxidation (fat burning) during high-intensity exercise like interval training or metabolic resistance training.

The Winner is: Pre-Workout Protein Smoothie

The nutrients you ingest around your workouts are extremely critical to developing and refining your physique. If you skip pre-workout protein, then you skip a chance to support intra-workout anabolism (muscle growth AND reduce post-workout catabolism (muscle breakdown).

Provided that you're getting adequate dietary protein throughout the day, I recommend BCAAs pre-workout. Their free form offers much faster absorption and uptake, which means your blood amino levels will be high when you hit the training floor.

Thank you Mike Rousell for your extensive and thought provoking research into this topic.

He can be contacted at drmike@mikeroussell.com

# ENERGY / PRE WORKOUT SMOOTHIES

**Strawberry, Banana & Grape Smoothie** ⊕

2 handfuls greens

1/2-cup water

2 bananas, peeled and frozen

½ cup red grapes

11/2 cups frozen strawberries

1 Scoop protein powder (Hemp protein)

**Minty pear Smoothie**

2 handfuls greens

1/2 cup water

2 pears cored

¼ inch section of fresh ginger, grated

¼ cup chopped fresh mint leaves - 1 Scoop protein powder (Hemp protein)

## Pear & Orange Smoothie

2 handfuls greens

½ cup ice

1 pear, cored and seeded

2 oranges, peeled and seeded

1 tablespoon of ground flaxseed

1 banana, peeled and frozen

1 Scoop protein powder (Hemp protein)

## Peach & Mango Smoothie

2 handfuls greens

1 - cup water

11/2 cups frozen peaches

2 nectarines, peeled, cored and seeded

1 - cup frozen mango chunks

2 plums, cored and seeded

1 Scoop protein powder (Hemp protein)

## Coconut & Berries Smoothie

2 handfuls greens

1 - cup water

2 nectarines, peeled, cored, and seeded

1 banana, peeled and frozen

½ cup goji berries

½ cup shredded coconut

1 Scoop protein powder (Hemp protein)

# HEALTHY HEART SMOOTHIES

**Banana & Mango Smoothie**

2 handfuls greens

2 cups water

1 banana, peeled and frozen

¼ cup frozen mango chunks

2 teaspoons spirulina

2 tablespoons walnut oil

**Banana & Almond Smoothie**

2 handfuls greens

11/2 cups almond milk

3 bananas, peeled and frozen - ½ teaspoon cinnamon

124

**Coconut & Berry Smoothie**

2 handfuls greens

1-cup water

1 - cup frozen blueberries

¼ cup goji berries


**Watermelon & Mint Smoothie**

2 handfuls greens

4 cups watermelon

2 tablespoons ground flaxseeds


**Orange & Sunflower Smoothie**

2 handfuls greens

1-cup water

2 oranges, peeled and seeded

1 - cup red grapes

2 tablespoons ground flaxseed

2 tablespoons sunflower oil


125

**Avocado & Apple Smoothie**

2 handfuls greens

1 - cup unsweetened apple juice

1-cup ice

2 small apples, cored and seeded

½ avocado, peeled and cored

½ cup beets, peeled and diced -1-tablespoon cacao powder


**Peach & Berry Smoothie**

2 handfuls greens

1-cup water

11/2 cups frozen peaches

1 - cup mixed berries

1/2 avocado, peeled and cored


**Pear & Banana Smoothie**

2 handfuls greens

11/2 cups almond milk

2 pears cored

1 banana, peeled and frozen - ½ teaspoon vanilla extract


126

# BOOSTING YOUR IMMUNITY

**Blueberry Smoothie with Artichoke**

Half cup of blueberries

Half cup of your favourite yogurt

Half a cup of ice

Half a banana

1 Tablespoon Raw Organic Jerusalem artichoke Powder

**Cantaloupe & Carrot Smoothie**

2 handfuls greens

1/2-cup green tea

1 banana, peeled and frozen

1 carrot, chopped

1 - cup cantaloupe, peeled, seeded, and chopped

1 packet stevia / .

**Strawberry & Green Smoothie ⊕**

2 handfuls greens

1/2-cup green tea

½ cups frozen strawberries

1 banana, peeled and frozen

1 packet stevia

**Strawberry & Orange Smoothie**

2 handfuls greens

1/2-cup water

2 cups frozen strawberries

1 large orange, peeled and seeded

1 packet stevia.

**Blackberry & Mango Smoothie**

2 handfuls greens

1-cup water

½ cup frozen blackberries

½ cup frozen raspberries

1 - cup frozen mango chunks

1 orange, peeled and seeded

1 packet stevia

**Banana & Lemon Smoothie**

2 handfuls greens

1-cup ice

1 banana, peeled and frozen

½ cup green grapes

1 lemon, seeded and peeled

1 packet stevia.

# STRESS BEATER SMOOTHIES

**Apple & Banana Smoothie ⊕**

2 cups water

2 handfuls greens

2 small apples, cored and seeded

2 bananas, peeled and frozen

1 pear, seeded

1-tablespoon ground chia seed

**Pomegranate & Berry Smoothie ⊕**

2 handfuls greens

129

½ cup pomegranate juice

1 banana, peeled and frozen

½ cup frozen blueberries

½ cup strawberries

½ cup red grapes


**Pineapple & Greens Smoothie**

2 handfuls greens

1-cup water

2 cups pineapple chunks

1 - cup frozen peaches

1 banana, peeled and frozen


**Grapefruit, Kiwi & Banana Smoothie**

2 handfuls greens

1-cup coconut water

1 pink grapefruit, peeled and seeded

2 kiwis (skin on)

1 banana, peeled and frozen


130

# FAT BURNING SMOOTHIES

### The Fat-Burner Smoothie

2 handfuls greens

2 cups cooled green tea

½ can coconut milk

Juice of 1 lemon

¼ cup pitted dates

½ avocado, peeled and pitted

½ grapefruit, peeled and seeded


### Orange & Banana Green Smoothie

2 handfuls greens

½ cup water

2 oranges, peeled and seeded

2 bananas, peeled and frozen


### Very Pear & Berry Smoothie

2 handfuls greens

11/2 cups almond milk

2 cups frozen mixed berries - 2 pears, seeded

## Banana, Berry &Almond Smoothie ⊕

2 handfuls greens

11/2 cups Almond milk

1 banana, peeled and frozen

1 - cup frozen blueberries

½ cup frozen strawberries


## Strawberry & Cantaloupe Smoothie

2 handfuls greens

1-cup water

½ cantaloupe, peeled and seeded

11/2 cups frozen strawberries


## Cherry & Orange Smoothie

2 handfuls greens

11/2 cups almond milk

1-cup cherries, pitted

2 oranges, peeled and seeded

1-tablespoon chia seeds

## Raspberry & Orange Smoothie

2 handfuls greens

½ cup water

2 oranges, peeled and seeded

2 cups frozen raspberries

## The Peachy Vanilla Smoothie

2 handfuls greens

1-cup water

11/2 cups frozen peaches

1 - cup frozen strawberries

1-teaspoon vanilla extract

## Orange, Mango & Lime Smoothie

2 handfuls greens

11/2 cups water

1 orange, peeled and seeded

½ cup frozen mango chunks

1 lime, peeled and seeded

1 packet stevia.

## The Green Raspberry Smoothie ⊕

2 handfuls greens

1-cup water

1 banana, peeled and frozen

1 - cup frozen raspberries

2 tablespoons ground flaxseed

## Banana & Pear Smoothie

2 handfuls greens

11/2 cups water

1 banana, peeled and frozen

2 pears cored and seeded

2 tablespoons ground chia seed

## Pineapple & Orange Smoothie

2 handfuls greens

1-cup ice

1-cup pineapples chunks

2 oranges, peeled and seeded

134

**Watermelon & Seed Smoothie**

2 handfuls greens

1-cup ice

2 cups watermelon

1-teaspoon ground flaxseeds

**Grapefruit & Pineapple Smoothie**

2 handfuls greens

1/2-cup coconut water

½ cup ice

1-cup pineapple chunks

1 pink grapefruit

# MOOD ENHANCING SMOOTHIES

**Walnut & Mango Smoothie**

2 handfuls greens

11/2 cups almond milk

11/2 cups frozen mango chunks

1 banana, peeled and frozen - 1 tablespoon walnut oil

## Banana & Nectarine Smoothie ⊕

2 handfuls greens

1-cup water

2 bananas, peeled and frozen

1 nectarine, peeled and pitted

1 - cup frozen strawberries

3-pitted dates

## Red Berry Medley smoothie

2 handfuls greens

1-cup water

2 small red apples, cored and seeded

1 - cup frozen strawberries

## Berry Medley & Banana Smoothie

2 handfuls greens

11/2 cups water

1 banana, peeled and frozen

2 cups frozen mixed berries

2 tablespoons ground flaxseeds

136

**Papaya & Pineapple Smoothie**

2 handfuls greens

1/2-cup ice

1 papaya, peeled and seeded

11/4 cups fresh pineapple chunks


**Banana & Coconut Smoothie**

2 handfuls greens

1/2-cup ice

2 bananas, peeled and frozen

1 lime, peeled and seeded

½ cup shredded coconut

¼ cup fresh chopped coconut

1-cup coconut water - ½ avocado, peeled and pitted


**Blueberry & Beets Smoothie**

2 handfuls greens

1 - cup water

1 Banana, peeled and frozen

11/2 cups frozen peaches

1 - cup frozen blueberries

½ beet, peeled and diced

1 carrot, chopped

**Avocado & Banana Smoothie**

2 handfuls greens

1 - cup water

2 oranges, peeled and seeded

1 banana, peeled and frozen

½ avocado, peeled and pitted

**Pear & Vanilla Smoothie**

2 handfuls greens

1 - cup almond milk

½ cup ice

1 apple

1 banana, peeled and frozen

1 pear

2 tablespoons ground flaxseeds

1-teaspoon vanilla extract

# PREGNANCY / KID FRIENDLY SMOOTHIES

### Orange, Almond & Apricot Smoothie ⊕

2 handfuls greens

1 - cup water

2 oranges, peeled and seeded

6 dried apricots, pitted

1 banana, peeled and frozen

½ cup almonds

½ cup almond butter

### Blueberry & Banana Smoothie

2 handfuls greens

1 - cup water

1 large banana, peeled and frozen

11/4 cups frozen blueberries

¼ cup ground flaxseeds

1 packet stevia

### Chocolate Nut Smoothie

2 handfuls greens

139

2 cups water

½ cup cashew nuts

½ cup raw cacao powder

6 large pitted dates

1 packet stevia.


**Chocolate & Banana Smoothie**

2 handfuls greens

11/2 cups water

2 bananas, peeled and frozen

1 - cup hazelnut butter

4 large pitted dates

¼ cup raw cacao powder


**Black n Blueberry Almond Smoothie**

1-handful greens

2 cups almond milk

1 banana, peeled and frozen

½ cup frozen blueberries

1 - cup frozen blackberries - 2 pitted dates

**Berry-Berry Almond Smoothie**

2 handfuls greens

11/2 cups almond milk

2 teaspoons fresh lemon juice

2 cups frozen mixed berries

¼ cup goji berries

6 large pitted dates

1 packet stevia.


**The Berry Medley Smoothie**

1-handful greens

11/2 cups cashew milk

21/2 cups frozen mixed berries

4 large pitted dates

2 teaspoons vanilla extract


**Orange & Apricot Smoothie**

2 handfuls greens

1 - cup water

2 oranges, peeled and seeded

6 dried apricots, pitted

1 banana, peeled and frozen

½ cup almonds

¼ cup almond butter

**Berry & Banana Smoothie**

2 handfuls greens

1 - cup water

1 large banana, peeled and frozen

11/4 cups frozen blueberries

¼ cup ground flaxseed

1 packet stevia.

**Chocolate & Nut Smoothie**

2 handfuls greens

2 cups water

½ cup cashew nuts

½ cup raw cacao powder

6 large pitted dates

1 packet stevia.

## Chocolate & Banana Smoothie

2 handfuls greens

11/2 cups water

2 bananas, peeled and frozen

1 - cup hazelnut butter

4 large pitted dates

¼ cup raw cacao powder


## Blackberry & Almond Smoothie

2 handfuls greens

2 cups almond milk

1 banana, peeled and frozen

½ cup frozen blueberries

1 - cup frozen blackberries

2 pitted dates


## Berry almond

2 handfuls greens

11/2 cups almond milk

2 teaspoons fresh lemon juice


143

2 cups of frozen mixed berries

¼ cup goji berries

6 large pitted dates

1 packet stevia


**Berry Medley**

2 handfuls greens

11/2 cups cashew milk

21/1 - cups frozen mixed berries

4 large pitted dates

2 teaspoons vanilla extract


# CONSTIPATION SMOOTHIES

**Beet Pears**

2 handfuls greens

11/2 cups almond milk

2 large pears

¼ cup beets. Peeled and diced

**Banana Blueberry**

2 handfuls greens

1 - cup water

1 pear

1 banana, peeled and frozen

**Banana Prunes**

2 handfuls greens

11/2 cups almond milk

2 banana, peeled and frozen

5 prunes, seeded

1 pear

**Orange Mango**

2 handfuls greens

1 - cup water

1 - cup frozen mango chunks

2 oranges, peeled and seeded

**Strawberry Kiwi**

2 handfuls greens

1 - cup water

11/2 cups frozen strawberries

2 kiwis (skin on)

2 tablespoons flaxseeds

# HEALING SMOOTHIES FOR STRONG BONES & JOINTS

**Banana Berry**

2 handfuls greens

2 cups water

1 - cup frozen blueberries

1 banana, peeled

2 tablespoons ground chi seeds

**Banana Nut**

2 handfuls greens

1 - cup almond milk

2 bananas, peeled and frozen

146

2 tablespoons cacao

2 tablespoons ground flaxseed

## Lemon Zest

2 handfuls greens

11/2 cups fresh-squeezed orange juice

1 - cup ice

1 lemon, peeled

1 tablespoon MSM powder

## Ginger Pear

2 handfuls greens

1 - cup almond milk

2 large pears

1 inch ginger peeled

## Orange Avocado

2 handfuls greens

1 - cup water

½ cup ice

3 oranges peeled

½ avocado peeled and pitted

2 teaspoons Spirulina Powder

# ANTI-AGING SMOOTHIES.

**Watermelon Ginger Greens**

2 handfuls greens

½ cup ice

4 cups water melon chunks

2 tablespoons chia seeds

1 inch fresh ginger

**Banana Nut Greens**

2 handfuls greens

11/2 cups almond milk

3 bananas, peeled

2 tablespoons chia seeds

**Berry Coconut**

2 handfuls greens

148

11/2 cups coconut water

½ cup frozen blueberries

½ cup frozen raspberries


**Peach banana greens**

2 handfuls greens

2 cups water

11/2 cups frozen peaches

1 banana peeled

2 tablespoons sunflower oil

2 teaspoons Spirulina


# BEAUTY SMOOTHIES FOR VIBRANT SKIN, HAIR AND NAILS

**Cucumber Strawberry**

2 handfuls greens

1 - cup water

1 cucumber

1 - cup frozen strawberries

4 dried figs

2 tablespoons ground flaxseed

11/2 cups frozen mango chunks

**Mango Banana**

2 handfuls greens

1 - cup coconut water

1 banana, peeled

11/2 cups frozen mango chunks

**Papaya Lemon**

1 handful parsley

2 cups water

1 banana, peeled and frozen

1 - cup papaya chunks

1 lemon peeled

**Orange spinach**

2 cups of baby spinach

1 orange, peeled and seeded

1 kiwi, peeled

150

1 tablespoon apple cider vinegar

1 packet stevia

**Banana Pear**

2 handfuls greens

11/2 cups water

1 banana, peeled and frozen

2 pears

1/3 cup almond butter

**Apple Pear**

2 handfuls greens

2 stalks celery, chopped

½ cup water

1 pear, seeded

1 large apple, **cored**

1 banana frozen

2 tablespoons fresh lemon juice

**Green Berry**

2 handfuls greens

½ cup water

½ cup green tea

2 cups mixed berries

1 banana frozen


**Carrot Apple**

2 handfuls greens

3 stalks celery

1 - cup water

1 small beet, peeled and diced

1 - cup ice

2 carrots

1 apple

½ lemon, seeded, peeled and sectioned


**Cranberry Berry**

2 handfuls greens

½ cup ice

½ cup blueberries

½ cup blackberries

½ cup cranberries

1 tablespoon ground chia seeds

# CHAPTER 8

## WHY SHOULD I BUY ORGANIC?

The dirty dozen and clean 15.

A new report recommended eating produce without toxic pesticides would reduce your risk of getting cancer and other diseases. According to an organization of scientists, researchers and policymakers, certain types of organic produce can reduce the amount of toxins you consume on a daily basis by as much as 80 %.

Here I have put together two lists, "The Dirty Dozen" and the "Clean 15" to help you know when to buy organic and when it will not be necessary. I have compiled this lists using data from the USDA on the amount of pesticide residue found in non-organic fruits and vegetables after they had been washed.

The fruits and vegetables on "The Dirty Dozen" list, when conventionally grown, tested positive for at least 47 different chemicals, with some testing positive for up to 67. For produce on the "dirty" list, you should definitely try and go organic

The Dirty Dozen" list includes:

- Celery

- Peaches

- Strawberries

- Apples

- Domestic blueberries

- Nectarines

- Sweet bell peppers

- Spinach, kale and collard greens

- Cherries

- Potatoes

- Imported grapes

- Lettuce

All the produce on *The Clean 15* bore little to no traces of pesticides, and is safe to consume in non-organic form. This list includes:

- Onions

- Avocados

- Sweet corn

- Pineapples

- Sweet peas

- Asparagus

- Kiwi fruit

- Cabbage

- Eggplant

- Cantaloupe

156

- Watermelon

- Grapefruit

- Sweet potatoes

- Sweet onions

Why are some types of produce more prone to sucking up pesticides than others? A senior vice president of policy for the Environmental Working Group Richard Wiles says, *"If you eat something like a pineapple or sweet corn, they have a protection defense because of the outer layer of skin. Not the same for strawberries and berries."*

The President's Cancer Panel recommends washing conventionally grown produce to remove residues. Wiles adds, *"You should do what you can do, but the idea you are going to wash pesticides off is a fantasy. However, you should still wash them because you will reduce pesticide exposure."*

# Chapter 9

## Warm / Winter Soup Cleanse recipes.

## Highly energising Soup

Serves 2

This is definitely a highly energizing soup and is a big favourite while on a detox diet. Contains avocado that is high in EFAs and cucumber that is well known for its cleansing properties. The taste of this soup can be dramatically altered by the use of the herbs and spices mentioned or by alternating between the lemon and lime.

1 Avocado

2 Spring onions

1/2 Red or green pepper

1 Cucumber

2 Handfuls of spinach

1/2 clove of garlic

100ml of light vegetable Bouillon (yeast free)

Juice of 1 lemon or lime

Optional: coriander, parsley, and cumin.

Blend the avocado and stock to form a light paste and then add the other ingredients and BLEND. Now warm and enjoy.

# WARM BROCCOLI SOUP

Serves 2

This is definitely a winter favourite and destroys the myth that all raw food has to be cold and unwelcoming! By steaming the broccoli for just 5-6 minutes, the meal remains raw, but gains enough warmth to give that filling comforting feeling of soup. The texture given by the broccoli and the kick of the ginger makes this an excellent choice.

1/2 Avocado

6 -8 decent size broccoli heads

1/3 Red Onion

1 Celery Stick

Big Handful of Spinach

An Inch of Root Ginger

Cumin (Optional)

Lightly steam the broccoli (5-6 minutes) and put with all ingredients in a blender. Add garlic, pepper, and real salt to taste. The heat from the broccoli makes this deliciously gentle warm soup for winter.

# Autumn Tomato & Avocado Soup

Serves 2

This is a nice soup to have either cold (a bit like gazpacho) or warmed (on a slightly chilly morning or evening)

5 Large ripe, (preferably vine) tomatoes.

1 Ripe avocado

1 Spring onion

1/4 Cup ground almonds (freshly done yourself, not packet)

1-cup broth from Swiss Vegetable Bouillon

1/4 Teaspoon dill seed

Dash cayenne pepper

Add sea salt & cracked black pepper to taste.

All you need to do is place all of the ingredients into a blender (except one of the tomatoes) and blend! Depending on whether you are going cold or warm - then place the soup into a pan and warm very slightly. Warming but don't boil or cook (not painful to put your finger into) still means that the soup is raw. Add the last tomato (sliced) on top and serve.

A GUT FELLING PROBIOTIC SMOOTHIES.

# CHAPTER 10

## WHICH BLENDER?

What do I need form my blender?

**Review of the top 5 blenders from counter top to personal and even 'on the go' blenders.**

Amazon have a full range of blenders even if you don't buy from them, look at their range and customer reviews to help choose the best blender for YOU.

Most households have a blender so you can start with this and make some of the recipes, but read on. You will end up using this everyday so convenience is a huge factor when buying. So read on and find out some blender options then you can really start you healthy smoothie diet.

**Essential, A tight-fitting lid.** Following a in-depth consumer report there were more than a few blenders that were downgraded in professional tests because of splattering and spills. Additionally, the appliance lid should have a removable plug for adding liquids, and be easy to put on and take off. Pour spouts in lids are useful can make it easier to transfer ingredients.

**A stable base.** Blenders that feel wobbly or vibrate a lot when they blend are likely not performing at peak efficiency, which means they can take longer to blend.

**Easy cleanup.** Some blenders reviewed require a whirl of soapy water in the pitcher immediately after using, while others can be loaded straight into the dishwasher. Shy away from jars that have to be hand washed -- you're in danger of cuts from the sharp blades if they are not removable.

**Versatility.** If you only want a blender to make smoothies, or to perform other single tasks, stick with a less expensive blender with just a few settings, but if you want one that can perform a wide variety of blending, mixing and chopping jobs, buy the best blender for your money.

**A good warranty.** Because blenders take such a heavy beating, the standard one-year warranty is a must, but heavy-duty blenders carry much longer and more appealing warranties. Some experts say that the longer warranty is worth the extra money.

**How will you use the blender?** If you're looking to blend basic smoothies and shakes, there's no need to invest in a heavy-duty blender. Stick with less expensive, single-serve blender, or buy a cheap full-size blender, there are plenty out there. If you want to do a variety of tasks, and perhaps save having to buy another tool to do them, buy the best general use blender you can. These can generally run between $100 and $200. If you're a serious from-scratch baker and want to make your own flours and nut butters, a heavy-duty blender, usually around $400 and up, will be your best kitchen friend.

**Are you blending for one -- or two?** Full-size blenders can hold anywhere from 5 to 9 cups. They're great for families or if you often blend drinks at parties. Single-serve blenders hold 2 cups or less, plenty if you want to blend one shake -- and you can drink straight from the blending jar, so there's less cleanup.

Convenience is essential, this has got to be easy to transition from your regular breakfast and meal eating habits to easily using your smoothie maker.

**How often will you use it?** If you plan to blend the occasional milkshake or batch of soup, reviews say a good, inexpensive blender will suit you well. But if you're an avid cook or you blend multiple smoothies per day, you'll be better off with a sturdier, more powerful blender.

164

**Where will you store it?** Yes, consider that something used every day and first thing in the morning will have to either be a counter top position or easily stored in your cupboard above/below your counter. Also consider the weight if you plan to store the blender in a cabinet; heavy blenders can be a chore to wrangle from an upper shelf, or lift from a lower cabinet.

The standard space between a kitchen countertop and the cabinets above is 18 inches. Most blenders are designed to be shorter than this, so they'll fit neatly on the back of the counter -- but some are taller, notably the 20.5-inch for example Vitamix 5200.

**Does your blender need to match your décor?** Really.. Ok! If so, then color is a consideration for you, especially if you plan to store the blender on your countertop. Many blenders come in black or brushed-metal finish, while some manufacturers offer a rainbow of colors.

**Do you want the bonus features?** Some extras add convenience and save time: a lid with a removable plug for adding ingredients while blending, and pre-programmed settings, such as "ice crush" or "smoothie," let you press one button and walk away -- the blender will run the cycle and stop itself.

# MY TOP 5 BLENDERS.

1.

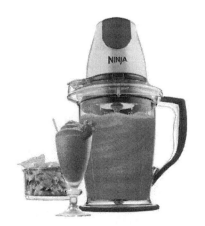

## Ninja Master Prep With Patented Blade Technology

Putting the power literally in the palm of your hand with the Ninja Master Prep. Crush ice into snow in seconds, blends frozen fruits into creamy smoothies, and even chops fresh ingredients quite evenly! This is a number! Best seller and no wonder it also does Mince, dice, chop, blend, and puree for consistent results in the 16 oz (2 cup) chopper bowl and achieve perfect frozen blending in the 48 oz (6 cup) pitcher. **From $30.00** a great smoothie blender

2.

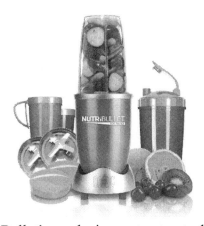

## Ninja Master Prep (QB900B) This Nutri-Bullet System is one of the best products out there to make healthy, nutritious drinks that can help you fight and prevent disease, lose weight, relieve joint pain, promote healthy, younger-looking skin, and even add years to your life. The Bullet's exclusive extractor technology uses a 600 watt motor

with cyclonic action and the patented extractor blades. This technology breaks down and pulverizes the stems, seeds, and skins where most of the essential nutrition lies – unlike what juicers and blenders do. One of the best part is a Nutri-Blast takes only seconds to prepare, seconds to clean and couldn't be easier to take on-the-go. **From $80.00** a great smoothie blender

3.

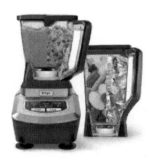

### Ninja Kitchen System 1200 (BL700) The Ninja Kitchen System 1200 is equipped with 1100 watts of professional power for all of your dough making, food processing and blending needs. This professional kitchen system offers a wide range of versatility, allowing you to KNEAD dough into creative pizzas, pretzels, breads and cookies, CRUSH ice into snow in seconds, BLEND whole fruits & veggies into delicious smoothies or use the PULSE button for controlled processing. **From $100.00** + this is a great smoothie blender and currently the one I use.

4.

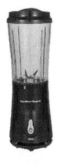

### Hamilton Beach 51101B Personal Blender with Travel Lid This is a compact design ideal for small living spaces and especially on-the-go

portability. It is great for making smoothies, shakes, baby formula, marinades and salad dressings Efficient 175-watt motor provides all the power you need for fast, reliable performance with a 14-oz. blending jar Also functions as portable travel cup that fits most car drink holders BPA free in food zones. The drinking lid with spout allows for easy sipping A durable, stainless steel cutting blades easily blend smoothies and shakes using either frozen or fresh fruit in the mixture Sturdy base rests on any surface. A simple one-touch operation with ON/PULSE button Jar and lid are dishwasher safe. **From $15.00** a great smoothie blender for on the go.

5.

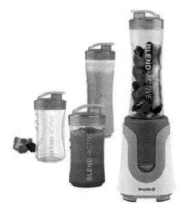

## Breville Blend-Active Personal Blender Family Pack

Ideal for the gym, work, school and days out - Just Blend & Go WITH one-touch blending for smoothies, shakes, slushies, and protein drinks 2 x 600ml and 2 x 300ml BPA-free bottles for all the family Detachable dishwasher-safe blades and bottle 300w motor useful "To-Go" cups. From just 30.00 GBP. The US / International Similar version is named **OSTER** For an overall great smoothie blender.

# CONGRATULATIONS

Well we're nearly at the end of my book, by this point I hope you have enjoyed many different recipes and are feeling healthier and happier.

So tell me what did you think? Did I really help you? How can I improve and get better? Please email me and let me know… I do hope you agreed that there were some amazing recipes. Smoothies and healthy information, all you need to start a healthy Smoothie diet.

I am continuously researching and improving my books, I want to provide you with the latest and best information.

Follow me on Real Healthy Kinda Food on FACEBOOK For the latest healthy recipes, information and just real healthy Kinda living".

…"I really can't wait to hear some of your real life stories and learn of your creative smoothie recipes. I also look forward to receiving your feed back on how much you and your whole family benefit from the healthy smoothies.

I sincerely hope I meet your satisfaction after you start this amazing healthy diet".

Oliver Michaels:

## Medical Disclaimer.

This book is not designed to, and does not provide medical advice. All content ("content"), including text, graphics, images and information available on or throughout this book are for general informational purposes only gained through the authors extensive research and experiences.

The content is not intended to be a substitute for professional medical advice, diagnosis or treatment. Never disregard professional medical advice, or delay in seeking it, because of something you have read in this book. Never rely on information in this book in place of seeking professional medical advice.

A gut feeling. Probiotic smoothies author is not responsible or liable for any advice, course of treatment, diagnosis or any other information, services or products that you obtain through this book. You are encouraged to confer with your doctor with regard to information contained in or through this book. After reading the content from this book, you are encouraged to review the information carefully with your professional healthcare provider.

CLEANSE-HEAL-ENERGISE & LOSE WEIGHT

Printed in Great Britain
by Amazon